Practitioner's Guide
to Symptom Base Rates
in the General Population

Practitioner's Guide
to Symptom Base Rates
in the General Population

Robert J. McCaffrey
Lyndsey Bauer
Sid E. O'Bryant
Anjali A. Palav

Editors

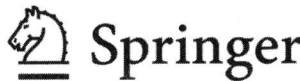 Springer

Robert J. McCaffrey
Lyndsey Bauer
and
Anjali A. Pavlav
Department of Psychology
State University of New York at Albany
Albany, NY 12222
USA

Sid E. O'Bryant
New Orleans VA Medical Center
New Orleans, LA 70112-1262
USA

Library of Congress Control Number: 2005928174

ISBN-10: 0-387-26757-3   e-ISBN 0-387-26758-1
ISBN-13: 978-0387-26757-9

Printed on acid-free paper.

Printed in the United States of America.   (SPI/EB)

9 8 7 6 5 4 3 2 1

springeronline.com

To Antonio E. Puente, Ph.D., for a decade of labor and persistence on behalf of professional neuropsychology. Psychology owes you a debt that it will never be able to repay fully.

RJM

Thanks to Bob for providing the opportunity to work on this project. Sid, Anjali, and Matt, thank you for the time and effort you put into this project. Thanks to Josh and my parents for encouraging me through the process.

LB

To my wife, Leigh, thank you for your unwavering support. I would also like to thank Lyndsey, Bob, Anjali, Matt, and everyone else who made this project possible.

SEO

Contents

I / A Brief Overview of Base Rates

The term "base rate" refers to the "prevalence of an event, such as a symptom, sign, or disorder, within a given population" (McCaffrey, Palav, O'Bryant, & Labarge, 2003, pg. 1). Meehl and Rosen (1955) first demonstrated the importance of base rates in psychological testing nearly 50 years ago. Since that time there has been a wealth of literature published regarding the importance of this information during clinical decision making. One reason base rates are so important is because in clinical practice, it is rarely the case that the probability of having certain conditions (e.g., depression, schizophrenia, PTSD, Alzheimer's dementia, malingering) when presenting with certain symptoms is equal for all of the patients seen. The likelihood that a person has a specific condition given certain symptoms fluctuates with a variety of factors such as age, gender, and race. The prevalence of dementia in individuals over the age of 85 ranges from 20% to 50% (Heilman & Valenstein, 2003); stated another way, one out of every five to every other person within the United States over the age of 85 suffers from some form of dementia. The prevalence of dementia in individuals under the age of 85 is different; notably, lower. Therefore, clinicians must use base rate information to determine the confidence they can have in diagnosing a particular patient with a specific condition given the symptoms they report. That is, without appropriate base rate estimates, clinicians cannot estimate their diagnostic accuracy. As Gouvier et al (2002) pointed out, "The effect of base rates operates to skew diagnostic accuracy in favor of predictions to the more prevalent category and to reduce accuracy to the less prevalent category" (pg. 377).

SYMPTOM BASE RATES, DISORDERS, AND CLINICAL DECISION MAKING

The previous volume, *Practitioners Guide to Symptom Base Rates in Clinical Neuropsychology*, explained how symptom base rates can be translated into the prevalence of certain disorders. If one symptom or a constellation of symptoms is pathognomonic of a particular disease or disorder, then the base rate of those symptoms may be used interchangeably as the prevalence of a condition in a specified population. If there exists a diagnostic instrument to assess for the condition in question, and the test's sensitivity and specificity can be calculated or are known, all of this information can be used to calculate its predictive value (for a comprehensive explanation of predictive values complete with calculations, refer to the previous volume). Since clinicians often utilize diagnostic instruments and base their decisions on the results, it would be extremely useful for them to be able to approximate how accurate a test is when "classifying" or "diagnosing" someone as having or not having a specific condition.

The applicability of the previous volume's information in this example only applies, of course, in the instances in which symptoms are pathognomonic for a particular disease or disorder, and if there is a diagnostic instrument to assess for having the condition. It is sometimes the case that patients present with more diffuse problems that could be symptoms of a host of different diseases or disorders. For example, "trouble walking" in the previous volume was a reported symptom of chronic fatigue syndrome, multiple sclerosis, traumatic brain injury, multiple personality disorder, panic disorder, and schizophrenia. In this example, the clinician could probably rule out some of the possible underlying causes for the symptom rather quickly based on their previous experience and judgment. However, they would not be able to calculate the predictive value of a diagnostic instrument, and certainly not for their clinical decision with this information.

BASE RATES AND DIFFERENTIAL DIAGNOSES

The base rate information supplied in the previous and the current volume is most critical during the interview process and for considering differential diagnoses. As noted above, clinicians are frequently faced with general, subjective complaints of patients (e.g., headache, shortness of breath, dizziness, nausea, weight gain) for which they have presented for examination. Patients want to know if there is something wrong with them, and they rely on the expert to determine if their symptoms are out of the ordinary given their current medical condition and history. Faced with a patient's concerns the clinician must make a "statistical decision" (either explicitly or implicitly) regarding the patient's presenting symptom(s) relative to the base rate of this symptom(s) in the population from which the particular patient comes. It is at this point that the current and previous reference books provide very useful information. With the information provided in these two volumes, practitioners can determine if, in fact, a presenting symptom(s) is out of the ordinary given the patient's characteristics, whether the presenting complaints are consistent with what is to be expected with certain syndromes, illnesses, and diseases, as well as determine what other syndromes, illnesses, and diseases should be explored given the entirety of the patients' presenting symptom cluster. Based on this knowledge the clinician can move forward by ruling in or out various diagnoses of conditions.

One example that clinicians, both physician and psychologist alike, might encounter in their practice is that of a female patient between the ages of 45 and 60 (Hartman, Kirchengast, Albrecht, Metka, & Huber, 1995) who presents complaining of hot flushes or hot flashes. While the first thought may be to immediately attribute the symptom to menopause, this in fact may *not* be correct. While hot flushes/hot flashes are certainly common symptoms of menopause (McCaffrey et al. 2003, pg. 108-118) and menopause is definitely part of the differential diagnosis, hot flushes/hot flashes are also frequent symptoms of other medical conditions, and may also occur in non-clinical populations. From the previous volume, one can see that hot flushes/hot flashes occur frequently in Cancer Treatments (Chemotherapy = 36.4%, Radiation Therapy = 64%), General Anxiety Disorder (37.3%), Panic Disorder (31.6-76.5%), as well as Depression (71%). The current volume indicates that among control groups, the reported occurrence of hot flushes/hot flashes ranges from 1% to 57%. Therefore, for this example, the clinician must consider several possible causes before coming to any conclusions as to the underlying etiology of the complaint. Given the sheer number of symptoms reported in control conditions in the current volume, and in medical conditions in the previous volume, these two compilations present clinicians with a large amount of information that will surely aid their ability to make differential diagnoses based on presenting symptom pictures.

SUMMARY

Meehl and Rosen (1955) first demonstrated the importance of base rates in psychological assessment nearly five decades ago. These authors stated, "The chief reason for our ignorance of the base rates is nothing more subtle than our failure to compute them" (pg. 213). Researchers continue to report that base rates are still largely being ignored (Duncan & Snow, 1987; Gouvier, Hayes, & Smiroldo, 1998). It is because of this gap in the literature that the current book *Practitioner's Guide to Symptom Base Rates in the General Population* and the previous book *Practitioner's Guide to Symptom Base Rates in Clinical Neuropsychology* (McCaffrey et al. 2003) were created. If the diagnostic accuracy of our clinical decision-making process and our testing instruments are to be estimated, we must calculate the base rates of the symptoms, disorders, and diseases we assess for on a regular basis.

It is hoped that the present book will aid neuropsychological practitioners and other health care professionals in the evaluation of the presenting complaints of their patients. Base rates are of utmost importance in the estimation of diagnostic accuracy of neuropsychological and psychological assessment, as well as any other form of testing, as well as in the interview and differential diagnostic process. It is hoped that these two volumes will encourage additional researchers to report base rate information as well as detailed information regarding the population from which this information was obtained. In order to estimate the accuracy of our clinical diagnoses/decisions that are made on a daily basis, we must understand the importance of base rate information and make every attempt to collect and report this data. Last, the current introduction is meant to provide a brief overview of base rates and their utility in clinical neuropsychology. If the reader wishes to gain more detailed understanding regarding base rates s/he is referred to *Practitioner's Guide to Symptom Base Rates in Clinical Neuropsychology* (McCaffrey, Palav, O'Bryant, & Labarge, 2003) as well as other sources (e.g., Gordon, 1977; Gouvier 1999, 2001; Meehl & Rosen, 1955).

Key for Using Tables

Gender: Males/Females
Age: Mean (Standard Deviation); Range
Race: Caucasian/African American/Hispanic/Asian
Native American/Other
Timeframe: timeframe of symptom report

SAMPLE TABLE CHARACTERISTICS

Schaughency, et al. (1994)
n = 943
Diagnostic Criteria:
Gender: 483/460
Age: 15
Race:
Population Setting: community
Nationality: New Zealand
Other Sample Characteristics:
Method of Reporting: self-report
Timeframe: current

II / Control Groups: Adult

COLLEGE STUDENTS

Machulda, et al. (1998)
n = 141
Diagnostic Criteria:
Gender: 49/92
Age: 20.7 (18-22)
Race: 268/88/66/7/0/9

Population Setting: college undergraduates
Nationality: US
Other Sample Characteristics:
Method of Reporting: self-report
Timeframe:

Symptom	%
anxiety	87
concentration difference	80
depression	71
disordered sleep	41
dizziness	19
fatigue	83

Symptom	%
headache	57
irritability	74
sensitive to light	26
sensitive to sound	16

Freeston, et al. (1996)
n = 583
Diagnostic Criteria:
Gender: 216/367
Age: 22.6 (4.6)
Race: 268/88/66/7/0/9

Population Setting: university undergraduates
Nationality: Canada
Other Sample Characteristics:
Method of Reporting: self-report
Timeframe:

Symptom	%
difficulty concentrating or mind going blank because of anxiety	16.5
dizziness or lightheadedness	7.0
dry mouth	6.5
easily fatigued	36.0
exaggerated startle response	12.7
feeling keyed up or on edge	23.5
flushes or chill	9.1
frequent urination	13.9
irritability	26.2

Symptom	%
muscle tension, aches, or soreness	17.3
nausea, diarrhea, or abdominal distress	9.4
palpitations or accelerated heart rate	17.8
restlessness	36.0
shortness of breath smothering sensation	8.1
sweating, cold/clammy hands	17.5
trembling, twitchy or feeling shaky	3.9

trouble falling or staying asleep	27.1

trouble swallowing or lump in throat	5.8

Wong, et al. (1994)
n = 88
Diagnostic Criteria:
Gender:
Age: 19.0 (2.9)
Race:

Population Setting: university undergraduates
Nationality: Canada
Other Sample Characteristics:
Method of Reporting: self-report
Timeframe: 6 months

Symptom	%
are often impatient	62.5
become tired very easily	63.6
have difficulty concentrating while reading	81.8
have lost sense of taste and/or smell	4.5
have trouble remembering things	46.6
lose way despite being there before	12.5

Symptom	%
often troubled by too much noise	35.2
suffer from dizziness	33.0
suffer from ringing in the ears	48.9
very easily affected by alcohol	25.0

COMBAT VETERANS

Litz, et al. (1992)
n = 18
Diagnostic Criteria: DSM-III-R
Gender: 18/0
Age: 40.0 (3.0)
Race:

Population Setting: PTSD center referrals
Nationality: US
Other Sample Characteristics:
Method of Reporting: self-report
Timeframe: current

Symptom	%
arrhythmia	5.9
backache	38.9
black out spells	5.6
blurred vision	5.6
butterflies	27.8
constipation	11.1
diarrhea	11.1

Symptom	%
dizziness	27.8
gas	27.8
headache	38.9
heart flutters	11.1
impotence	5.6
inorgasmia	5.6
muscle aches	22.2

nail biting	5.6
nausea	0.0
racing heart	0.0
rapid breathing	0.0

ringing in ears	5.6
sexual disinterest	11.8
shortness of breath	5.6
stomach cramps	16.7

COMMUNITY MEMBERS

Ohayon, et al. (1997)
n = 4,927
Diagnostic Criteria:
Gender: 2,078/2,894
Age: 15-100
Race:

Population Setting: community
Nationality: UK
Other Sample Characteristics:
Method of Reporting: telephone
survey
Timeframe: current

Symptom	%
breathing pauses	3.8
snoring	40.3

Symptom	%
snoring and breathing pauses	2.5

Ohayon, et al. (1997)
n = 859
Diagnostic Criteria:
Gender:
Age: 15-24
Race:

Population Setting: community
Nationality: UK
Other Sample Characteristics:
Method of Reporting: telephone
survey
Timeframe: current

Symptom	%
breathing pauses	2.5
snoring	23.1

Ohayon, et al. (1997)
n = 935
Diagnostic Criteria:
Gender:
Age: 25-34
Race:

Population Setting: community
Nationality: UK
Other Sample Characteristics:
Method of Reporting: telephone
survey
Timeframe: current

Symptom	%
breathing pauses	2.7
snoring	38.1

Ohayon, et al. (1997)
n = 856
Dïagnostic Criteria:
Gender:
Age: 35-44
Race:

Population Setting: community
Nationality: UK
Other Sample Characteristics:
Method of Reporting: telephone
survey
Timeframe: current

Symptom	%
breathing pauses	4.8
snoring	45.8

Ohayon, et al. (1997)
n = 711
Diagnostic Criteria:
Gender:
Age: 45-54
Race:

Population Setting: community
Nationality: UK
Other Sample Characteristics:
Method of Reporting: telephone
survey
Timeframe: current

Symptom	%
breathing pauses	4.6
snoring	53.5

Ohayon, et al. (1997)
n = 631
Diagnostic Criteria:
Gender:
Age: 55-64
Race:

Population Setting: community
Nationality: UK
Other Sample Characteristics:
Method of Reporting: telephone
survey
Timeframe: current

Symptom	%
breathing pauses	5.1
snoring	49.3

Ohayon, et al. (1997)
n = 980
Diagnostic Criteria:
Gender:
Age: 65+
Race:

Population Setting: community
Nationality: UK
Other Sample Characteristics:
Method of Reporting: telephone
survey
Timeframe: current

Symptom	%
breathing pauses	3.9
snoring	37.3

Kaye, et al. (1983)
n = 24
Diagnostic Criteria:
Gender: 10/14
Age: 54.8 (33-85)
Race: 12/12/0/0/0/0

Population Setting: outpatients
Nationality: US
Other Sample Characteristics:
Method of Reporting: self-report
Timeframe: current

Symptom	%
difficulty falling asleep	25
difficulty staying asleep	14

Symptom	%
waking up earlier than intended	22

Krieger, et al. (1993)
n = 86
Diagnostic Criteria:
Gender:
Age: 38.8 (1.0)
Race:

Population Setting: occupational
medicine clinic outpatients
Nationality: France
Other Sample Characteristics:
Method of Reporting: self-report
Timeframe: current

Symptom	%
nocturnal micturitions	25

Honsberg, et al. (1995)
n = 1476
Diagnostic Criteria:
Gender: 663/813
Age: 46.3
Race: 1476/0/0/0/0/0

Population Setting: community
Nationality: US
Other Sample Characteristics:
Method of Reporting: postal survey
Timeframe: current

Symptom	%
habitual snoring	10.7

Jennum, et al. (1994)
n = 1670
Diagnostic Criteria:
Gender: 1670/0
Age: 54-75
Race:

Population Setting: community
Nationality: Denmark
Other Sample Characteristics: snore
often or always

Method of Reporting: self-report   Timeframe: 1 year

Symptom	%
concentration problems	6.0
headache	56.1
headache with nausea and vision disturbance	5.6

Symptom	%
memory problems	9.8
morning headache	10.7

Jennum, et al. (1994)
n = 1653
Diagnostic Criteria:
Gender: 1653/0
Age: 53-75
Race:

Population Setting: community
Nationality: Denmark
Other Sample Characteristics:
Method of Reporting: self-report
Timeframe: 1 year

Symptom	%
concentration problems	5.4
headache	44.7
headache with nausea and vision disturbance	3.7

Symptom	%
memory problems	8.2
morning headache	8.2

Linna, et al. (1991)
n = 1101
Diagnostic Criteria:
Gender: 568/533
Age: 8
Race:

Population Setting: community
Nationality: Finland
Other Sample Characteristics:
Method of Reporting: parent-report
Timeframe:

Symptom	%
enuresis-frequently	1.5
enuresis-occasionally	7.1
frequent abdominal pain	2.4
frequent soiling	0.3

Symptom	%
occasional distress	43.5
occasional soiling	3.5
recurrent headache	2.8

Linna, et al. (1991)
n = 533
Diagnostic Criteria:
Gender: 0/533
Age: 8
Race:

Population Setting: community
Nationality: Finland
Other Sample Characteristics:
Method of Reporting: parent-report
Timeframe:

Symptom	%
enuresis-frequently	1.2
enuresis-occasionally	9.1

Symptom	%
recurrent headache	3.1

Linna, et al. (1991)
n = 568
Diagnostic Criteria:
Gender: 568/0
Age: 8
Race:

Population Setting: community
Nationality: Finland
Other Sample Characteristics:
Method of Reporting: parent-report
Timeframe:

Symptom	%
enuresis-frequently	1.8
enuresis-occasionally	5.0

Symptom	%
recurrent headache	2.5

Schvarcz, et al. (1996)
n = 210
Diagnostic Criteria:
Gender: 104/106
Age: 37.2(4.7)
Race:

Population Setting: community
Nationality: Sweden
Other Sample Characteristics:
Method of Reporting: postal survey
Timeframe: 3 months

Symptom	%
abdominal discomfort or pain at defecation	8.5
abdominal discomfort or pain relieved by defecation	12.1
abdominal distension	24.4
alternating diarrhea and constipation	6.7
black stools	3.0
blood stains in stools	3.0
borborygui	20.6
constipation	10.3
diarrhea	13.4
dysphagia	1.2
early satiety	6.1
eructations	10.9

Symptom	%
feeling of incomplete defecation	17.0
flatus	14.6
heartburn	23.0
loss of appetite	3.6
mucous stools	4.9
nausea	9.1
nightly urge of defecation	1.2
reflux episodes	10.3
retrosternal pain	12.1
uncomfortable feeling of fullness after meals	8.5
vomiting	3.0
weight loss	0.6

Thomsen (1993)
n = 488
Diagnostic Criteria:
Gender: 488/0
Age:
Race:

Population Setting: public school children
Nationality: Denmark
Other Sample Characteristics:
Method of Reporting: self-report
Timeframe:

Symptom	%
a bad conscience but no one else	36.5
angry if someone messes desk	83.2
at night, put things away just so	42.6
doing things in an exact manner	61.5
favorite or special number	28.3
frequently indecisive	61.1
fussy about hands	50.0
hate dirt and contamination	48.4
have to check several times	43.0
have to do certain things	43.4
lack of confiance (repetition)	54.1

Symptom	%
need to count several times	26.6
repeated thoughts or words	62.7
repetition until correct	34.4
something touched is spoiled	25.4
special number or words to avoid	17.2
spending extra time on homework	36.1
talk or move to avoid bad luck	27.5
trouble finishing schoolwork	42.2
worry about being clean enough	57.8

Thomsen (1993)
n = 544
Diagnostic Criteria:
Gender: 0/544
Age:
Race:

Population Setting: public school children
Nationality: Denmark
Other Sample Characteristics:
Method of Reporting: self-report
Timeframe:

Symptom	%
a bad conscience but no one else	39.0
angry if someone messes desk	84.2

Symptom	%
at night, put things away just so	44.5
doing things in an exact manner	58.8

favorite or special number	30.9
frequently indecisive	71.0
fussy about hands	61.0
hate dirt and contamination	59.6
have to check several times	45.2
have to do certain things	47.1
lack of confiance (repetition)	58.8
need to count several times	24.3
repeated thoughts or words	65.8
repetition until correct	32.7

something touched is spoiled	25.0
special number or words to avoid	24.3
spending extra time on homework	37.9
talk or move to avoid bad luck	34.2
trouble finishing schoolwork	38.6
worry about being clean enough	51.8

Valleni-Basile, et al. (1994)
n = 363
Diagnostic Criteria:
Gender: 165/198
Age: 7th-9th grade
Race: 276/87/0/0/0/0

Population Setting: public school children
Nationality: US
Other Sample Characteristics:
Method of Reporting: structured interview
Timeframe:

Symptom	%
checking obsessions	1.1
collecting obsessions	0.0
compulsions only	2.2
counting obsessions	0.3
obsessions (one or more types)	2.8

Symptom	%
obsessions and compulsions	0.0
obsessions only	2.8
touching obsessions	0.3
washing obsessions	0.3

Degonda, et al. (1993)
n = 491
Diagnostic Criteria:
Gender:
Age: 21
Race:

Population Setting: community
Nationality: Switzerland
Other Sample Characteristics:
Method of Reporting: semi-structured interview
Timeframe: 12 months

Symptom	%
compulsion to wash	1.2

Symptom	%

compulsions to check and control	12.1
feelings of anxiety when not giving in to compulsion	3.1
obsessive counting	1.6

obsessive melodies	3.1
obsessive thoughts	2.7
other compulsions	0.0

Degonda, et al. (1993)
n = 456
Diagnostic Criteria:
Gender:
Age: 23
Race:

Population Setting: community
Nationality: Switzerland
Other Sample Characteristics:
Method of Reporting: semi-structured interview
Timeframe: 12 months

Symptom	%
compulsion to wash	0.0
compulsions to check and control	5.1
feelings of anxiety when not giving in to compulsion	0.5

Symptom	%
obsessive counting	1.1
obsessive melodies	0.0
obsessive thoughts	1.1
other compulsions	2.2

Degonda, et al. (1993)
n = 457
Diagnostic Criteria:
Gender:
Age: 28
Race:

Population Setting: community
Nationality: Switzerland
Other Sample Characteristics:
Method of Reporting: semi-structured interview
Timeframe: 12 months

Symptom	%
compulsion to wash	0.5
compulsions to check and control	3.3
feelings of anxiety when not giving in to compulsion	0.3

Symptom	%
obsessive counting	0.6
obsessive melodies	0.0
obsessive thoughts	0.8
other compulsions	2.0

Degonda, et al. (1993)
n = 424
Diagnostic Criteria:
Gender:
Age: 30
Race:

Population Setting: community
Nationality: Switzerland
Other Sample Characteristics:
Method of Reporting: semi-structured interview
Timeframe: 12 months

Symptom	%
compulsion to wash	0.4
compulsions to check and control	10.5
feelings of anxiety when not giving in to compulsion	0.0

Symptom	%
obsessive counting	2.0
obsessive melodies	0.0
obsessive thoughts	1.2
other compulsions	3.9

Degonda, et al. (1993)
n = 535
Diagnostic Criteria:
Gender:
Age: 21-30
Race:

Population Setting: community
Nationality: Switzerland
Other Sample Characteristics:
Method of Reporting: semi-structured interview
Timeframe: lifetime

Symptom	%
suicide attempts	9

Isoaho, et al. (1995)
n = 183
Diagnostic Criteria:
Gender: 183/0
Age: 71.4 (5.9, 64-86)
Race:

Population Setting: community
Nationality: Finland
Other Sample Characteristics:
Method of Reporting: self-report
Timeframe: current

Symptom	%
confusion	21
constipation	14
crying spells	2
decreased appetite	43
decreased libido	27
dissatisfaction	25
diurnal variation	35
emptiness	40
fatigue	17
hopelessness	27
indecisiveness	27

Symptom	%
irritability	6
marital dissatisfaction	0
personal devaluation	39
psychomotor agitation	12
psychomotor retardation	26
sadness	7
sleep disturbance	27
suicidal rumination	2
tachycardia	10
weight loss	17

Isoaho, et al. (1995)   n = 63

Diagnostic Criteria:
Gender: 0/63
Age: 72.2 (5.4, 64-86)
Race:
Population Setting: community

Nationality: Finland
Other Sample Characteristics:
Method of Reporting: self-report
Timeframe: current

Symptom	%
confusion	16
constipation	19
crying spells	12
decreased appetite	32
decreased libido	29
dissatisfaction	20
diurnal variation	37
emptiness	40
fatigue	25
hopelessness	22

Symptom	%
indecisiveness	39
irritability	3
marital dissatisfaction	0
personal devaluation	35
psychomotor agitation	10
psychomotor retardation	19
sadness	8
sleep disturbance	34
suicidal rumination	3
tachycardia	14
weight loss	9

Bjornsson, et al. (1994)
n = 3,294
Diagnostic Criteria:
Gender:
Age: 20-44
Race:

Population Setting: community
Nationality: Sweden
Other Sample Characteristics:
Vasterbotten
Method of Reporting: postal survey
Timeframe: 12 months

Symptom	%
asthma attack	3.3
breathless while wheezing	11.2
current asthma medications	6.2
hay fever/allergic rhinitis	21.1
long-term cough	15.9
morning cough	12.2

Symptom	%
productive cough	19.6
wheezing	19.8
wheezing without cold	12.2
woken by attacks of breathlessness	4.3
woken by attacks of cough	26.9
woken by chest tightness	10.4

Bjornsson, et al. (1994)
n = 3,147
Diagnostic Criteria:
Gender:
Age: 20-44
Race:

Population Setting: community
Nationality: Sweden
Other Sample Characteristics:
Uppsala
Method of Reporting: postal survey
Timeframe: 12 months

Symptom	%
asthma attack	3.3
breathless while wheezing	10.3
current asthma medications	4.9
hay fever/allergic rhinitis	22.2
long-term cough	16.5
morning cough	11.2

Symptom	%
productive cough	18.3
wheezing	19.0
wheezing without cold	11.4
woken by attacks of breathlessness	5.0
woken by attacks of cough	25.4
woken by chest tightness	9.7

Bjornsson, et al. (1994)
n = 2,884
Diagnostic Criteria:
Gender:
Age: 20-44
Race:

Population Setting: community
Nationality: Sweden
Other Sample Characteristics:
Goteborg
Method of Reporting: postal survey
Timeframe: 12 months

Symptom	%
asthma attack	3.1
breathless while wheezing	12.4
current asthma medications	4.8
hay fever/allergic rhinitis	22.2
long-term cough	19.6
morning cough	15.9

Symptom	%
productive cough	22.2
wheezing	23.0
wheezing without cold	13.5
woken by attacks of breathlessness	7.2
woken by attacks of cough	28.5
woken by chest tightness	14.7

Bjornsson, et al. (1994)
n = 4,533
Diagnostic Criteria:
Gender:
Age: 20-44
Race:

Population Setting: community
Nationality: Sweden
Other Sample Characteristics:
lifetime nonsmokers
Method of Reporting: postal survey
Timeframe: 12 months

Symptom	%
asthma attack	3.4
breathless while wheezing	8.4
current asthma medications	5.4
hay fever/allergic rhinitis	23.4
long-term cough	13.9

Symptom	%
morning cough	6.9
productive cough	13.7
wheezing	14.6
wheezing without cold	8.8
woken by attacks of breathlessness	4.7

woken by attacks of cough	23.1

woken by chest tightness	9.2

Bjornsson, et al. (1994)
n = 1,473
Diagnostic Criteria:
Gender:
Age: 20-44
Race:

Population Setting: community
Nationality: Sweden
Other Sample Characteristics: ex-smokers
Method of Reporting: postal survey
Timeframe: 12 months

Symptom	%
asthma attack	3.2
breathless while wheezing	9.4
current asthma medications	6.2
hay fever/allergic rhinitis	22.5
long-term cough	14.4
morning cough	7.0
productive cough	14.7

Symptom	%
wheezing	16.5
wheezing without cold	8.1
woken by attacks of breathlessness	4.7
woken by attacks of cough	23.0
woken by chest tightness	11.0

Bjornsson, et al. (1994)
n = 3,319
Diagnostic Criteria:
Gender:
Age: 20-44
Race:

Population Setting: community
Nationality: Sweden
Other Sample Characteristics: current smokers
Method of Reporting: postal survey
Timeframe: 12 months

Symptom	%
asthma attack	3.1
breathless while wheezing	16.1
current asthma medications	4.9
hay fever/allergic rhinitis	19.0
long-term cough	22.9
morning cough	23.9
productive cough	30.6

Symptom	%
wheezing	30.6
wheezing without cold	19.1
woken by attacks of breathlessness	6.8
woken by attacks of cough	33.5
woken by chest tightness	15.0

Haraldsson, et al. (1992)
n = 112
Diagnostic Criteria:

Gender:
Age: 18-24
Race:

Population Setting: community
Nationality: Sweden
Other Sample Characteristics:

Method of Reporting: postal survey
Timeframe: current

Symptom	%
snoring	24.4
diurnal hypersomnia	9.1
breath cessations	3.8
difficulty maintaining sleep	27.4

Symptom	%
snoring, diurnal hypersomnia and sleep disturbance	2.2

Haraldsson, et al. (1992)
n = 607
Diagnostic Criteria:
Gender: 292/315
Age: 30-69
Race:

Population Setting: community
Nationality: Sweden
Other Sample Characteristics:
Method of Reporting: postal survey
Timeframe: current

Symptom	%
snoring, diurnal hypersomnia, and sleep disturbance	3.1
multiple sleep apnea and diurnal hypersomnia	1.5

Symptom	%
snoring and breath cessations	3.0
snoring and diurnal hypersomnia	5.1

Haraldsson, et al. (1992)
n = 292
Diagnostic Criteria:
Gender: 292/0
Age: 30-69
Race:

Population Setting: community
Nationality: Sweden
Other Sample Characteristics:
Method of Reporting: postal survey
Timeframe: current

Symptom	%
multiple sleep apnea and diurnal hypersomnia	2.8
snoring, diurnal hypersomnia, and sleep disturbance	5.5

Symptom	%
snoring and diurnal hypersomnia	8.2
snoring and breath cessations	4.8

Haraldsson, et al. (1992)
n = 315
Diagnostic Criteria:
Gender: 0/315
Age: 30-69
Race:

Population Setting: community
Nationality: Sweden
Other Sample Characteristics:
Method of Reporting: postal survey
Timeframe: current

Symptom	%
multiple sleep apnea and diurnal hypersomnia	0.3
snoring, diurnal hypersomnia, and sleep disturbance	1.0
snoring and breath cessations	1.3

Symptom	%
snoring and diurnal hypersomnia	2.2

Silverman, et al. (1992)
n = 62
Diagnostic Criteria:
Gender: 18/44
Age:
Race: 57/30/10/10/0/0

Population Setting: laboratory study
Nationality: US
Other Sample Characteristics:
Method of Reporting: self-report
Timeframe: 2 days

Symptom	%
moderate or severe	2

Kales, et al. (1984)
n = 100
Diagnostic Criteria:
Gender: 41/59
Age: 48.2 (1.5, 24-80)
Race:

Population Setting: community
Nationality: US
Other Sample Characteristics:
Method of Reporting: self-report
Timeframe: current

Symptom	%
attempts at suicide	3.0
depressed	2.0
diarrhea	9.6
headache	1.1
mind racing before sleep	15.0
palpitations	16.0

Symptom	%
stomach discomfort	3.2
tense/anxious before sleep	2.0
tiredness	12.8
weakness	3.2
woke up refreshed most mornings	89.4

Schwab, et al. (1979)
n = 1645
Diagnostic Criteria:
Gender: 910/735
Age: 41.0 (17-92)
Race: 1277/368/0/0/0/0

Population Setting: community
Nationality: US
Other Sample Characteristics:
Method of Reporting: structured
interview
Timeframe: 1 year

Symptom	%
constipation	26.5
diarrhea	15.3
headaches	46.7
indigestion	33.9
nervous stomach	22.7

Symptom	%
stomach aches	22.5
too heavy	28.0
too thin	7.6
weight fluctuates	3.7

Merikangas, et al. (1993)
n = 218
Diagnostic Criteria:
Gender: 0/218
Age: 20-30
Race: 1277/368/0/0/0/0
Population Setting: community

Nationality: Switzerland
Other Sample Characteristics: [1]pre-
menstrual, [2]during menstruation
Method of Reporting: semi-structured
interview
Timeframe: 1 year

Symptom	%
acne [2]	26.1
anxiety [2]	1.0
better mood [1]	2.3
bloating [2]	7.8
depressed mood [1]	18.8
depressed mood [2]	10.6
dizziness [2]	5.0
headache [2]	16.5
increased activity [2]	2.3
increased anxiety [1]	3.2
irritability [1]	30.7

Symptom	%
irritability [2]	19.7
lower back pain [2]	29.8
nervousness [2]	8.7
nervousness [1]	18.3
nervousness [1]	4.1
sweating [2]	14.7
tension [1]	17.9
tension [2]	2.3
unspecific pain [2]	36.2
vomiting [2]	2.3
weight pain [2]	12.8

Merikangas, et al. (1993)
n = 152
Diagnostic Criteria:
Gender: 0/152
Age: 20-30
Race: 1277/368/0/0/0/0

Population Setting: community
Nationality: Switzerland
Other Sample Characteristics:
Method of Reporting: semi-structured
interview
Timeframe: 1 year

Symptom	%
suicide attempts	9.9

Ramcharan, et al. (1992)
n = 383
Diagnostic Criteria:
Gender: 0/383
Age: 34.1 (26-35)
Race:

Population Setting: community
Nationality: Canada
Other Sample Characteristics:
menstrual
Method of Reporting: self-report
Timeframe: 1 day

Symptom	%
arousal	5.4
autonomic reactions	7.3
behavioral change	8.1
control	6.4

Symptom	%
impaired concentration	4.9
negative affect	4.2
pain	10.9
water retention	11.8

Ramcharan, et al. (1992)
n = 331
Diagnostic Criteria:
Gender: 0/331
Age: 33.6 (26-35)
Race:

Population Setting: community
Nationality: Canada
Other Sample Characteristics: post-
menstrual
Method of Reporting: self-report
Timeframe: 1 day

Symptom	%
arousal	10.3
autonomic reactions	4.8
behavioral change	5.9
control	5.6

Symptom	%
impaired concentration	3.7
negative affect	6.8
pain	6.4
water retention	2.1

Ramcharan, et al. (1992)
n = 330
Diagnostic Criteria:
Gender: 0/330
Age: 34.0 (26-35)
Race:

Population Setting: community
Nationality: Canada
Other Sample Characteristics: mid-
cycle
Method of Reporting: self-report
Timeframe: 1 day

Symptom	%
arousal	4.7

Symptom	%
autonomic reactions	4.3

behavioral change	7.2
control	3.4
impaired concentration	4.7
negative affect	4.0

pain	3.1
water retention	1.8

Ramcharan, et al. (1992)
n = 334
Diagnostic Criteria:
Gender: 0/334
Age: 34.2 (26-35)
Race:

Population Setting: community
Nationality: Canada
Other Sample Characteristics: early
premenstrual
Method of Reporting: self-report
Timeframe: 1 day

Symptom	%
arousal	10.6
autonomic reactions	3.3
behavioral change	6.0
control	3.9

Symptom	%
impaired concentration	3.3
negative affect	3.4
pain	4.2
water retention	3.6

Ramcharan, et al. (1992)
n = 341
Diagnostic Criteria:
Gender: 0/341
Age: 34 (26-35)
Race:

Population Setting: community
Nationality: Canada
Other Sample Characteristics:
premenstrual
Method of Reporting: self-report
Timeframe: 1 day

Symptom	%
arousal	5.5
autonomic reactions	6.2
behavioral change	9.0
control	5.4

Symptom	%
impaired concentration	4.8
negative affect	4.5
pain	5.1
water retention	12.2

Cirignotta, et al. (1989)
n = 1170
Diagnostic Criteria:
Gender: 1170/0
Age: 50.1 (11.7)
Race:

Population Setting: community
Nationality: Italy
Other Sample Characteristics:
Method of Reporting: postal survey
Timeframe:

Symptom	%
snored always	10.1

Cirignotta, et al. (1989)
n = 340
Diagnostic Criteria:
Gender: 340/0
Age: 50.8 (11.5)
Race:

Population Setting: community
Nationality: Italy
Other Sample Characteristics:
Method of Reporting: telephone
survey
Timeframe:

Symptom	%
every-night snoring	5.6

Rutter, et al. (1976)
n = 96
Diagnostic Criteria:
Gender: 96/0
Age: 14-15
Race:

Population Setting: community
Nationality: UK
Other Sample Characteristics:
Method of Reporting: [1]self-report,
[2]other-report
Timeframe:

Symptom	%
ideas of reference [1]	28.1
observed anxiety[2]	19.8
observed sadness [2]	12.5
often feels miserable or depressed [1]	20.8
reported misery [1]	41.7
self depreciation [1]	19.8

Symptom	%
suicidal ideas [1]	7.3
usually has a great difficulty falling asleep [1]	20.8
usually wakes unnecessarily in morning [1]	22.9

Rutter, et al. (1976)
n = 88
Diagnostic Criteria:
Gender: 0/88
Age: 14-15
Race:

Population Setting: community
Nationality: UK
Other Sample Characteristics:
Method of Reporting: [1]self-report,
[2]other-report
Timeframe:

Symptom	%
ideas of reference [1]	30.7
observed anxiety[2]	28.4
observed sadness [2]	14.8
often feels miserable or depressed [1]	23.0
reported misery [1]	47.7

Symptom	%
self depreciation [1]	23.0
suicidal ideas [1]	7.9
usually has a great difficulty falling asleep [1]	17.2

usually wakes unnecessarily in morning [1]	24.1

Schoenbach, et al. (1982)
n = 384
Diagnostic Criteria:
Gender: 176/208
Age: 12-15
Race: 253/131/0/0/0/0

Population Setting: public junior high school students
Nationality: US
Other Sample Characteristics:
Method of Reporting: self-report
Timeframe:

Symptom	%
blues	16
could not get going	19
crying spells	14
depressed	19
did not enjoy life	28
everything an effort	36
feel like a failure	10
not as good as others	39
not happy	28

Symptom	%
not hopeful	41
overate	27
poor appetite	14
restless sleep	21
sad	15
slept more than usual	24
trouble concentrating	30

Suris, et al. (1996)
n = 383
Diagnostic Criteria:
Gender: 0/383
Age: 16.1 (1.3, 14-19)
Race: 253/131/0/0/0/0

Population Setting: high school and vocational students
Nationality: Spain
Other Sample Characteristics:
Method of Reporting: self-report
Timeframe:

Symptom	%
bad mood	2.9
believing nothing amused them	2.6
emotional problems	15.4
feeling sad	8.7

Symptom	%
frequent crying	17.2
lack of appetite	38.0
sleeping problems	23.3
suicidal thoughts	8.9

Suris, et al. (1996)
n = 482
Diagnostic Criteria:
Gender: 482/0
Age: 16.0 (1.3, 14-19)
Race: 253/131/0/0/0/0

Population Setting: high school and vocational students
Nationality: Spain
Other Sample Characteristics:
Method of Reporting: self-report
Timeframe:

Symptom	%
bad mood	4.0
believing nothing amused them	3.1
emotional problems	7.3
feeling sad	8.5

Symptom	%
frequent crying	3.2
lack of appetite	18.8
sleeping problems	19.1
suicidal thoughts	9.9

Wiggins, et al. (1990)
n = 360
Diagnostic Criteria:
Gender: 360/0
Age: 16.0 (1.3, 14-19)
Race: 0/0/360/0/0/0
Population Setting: community

Nationality: US
Other Sample Characteristics:
Method of Reporting: [1]structured interview, [2]structured interview of spouse
Timeframe:

Symptom	%
during usual sleep: choke or struggle for breath [1]	3.2
during usual sleep: choke or struggle for breath [2]	6.9
during usual sleep: snore loudly [1]	33.8
during usual sleep: snore loudly [2]	43.0
during usual sleep: toss and turn frequently [1]	23.9
during usual sleep: toss and turn frequently [2]	21.6
fall asleep as automobile driver [1]	3.5
fall asleep as automobile driver [2]	2.3
fall asleep as automobile passenger [1]	8.0

Symptom	%
fall asleep as automobile passenger [2]	11.7
fall asleep at school or church [1]	5.6
fall asleep at school or church [2]	5.0
fall asleep at work [1]	3.0
fall asleep at work [2]	1.2
fall asleep reading or watching TV [1]	24.6
fall asleep reading or watching TV [2]	35.0
fall asleep: after a meal [1]	20.1
fall asleep: after a meal [2]	26.3

Wiggins, et al. (1990)
n = 360
Diagnostic Criteria:
Gender: 0/360
Age: 16.0 (1.3, 14-19)

Race: 0/0/360/0/0/0
Population Setting: community
Nationality: US
Other Sample Characteristics:

Method of Reporting: [1]structured
interview, [2]structured interview of

spouse
Timeframe:

Symptom	%
during usual sleep: choke or struggle for breath [1]	3.4
during usual sleep: choke or struggle for breath [2]	2.9
during usual sleep: snore loudly [1]	18.4
during usual sleep: snore loudly [2]	17.4
during usual sleep: toss and turn frequently [1]	25.9
during usual sleep: toss and turn frequently [2]	13.3
fall asleep as automobile driver [1]	2.1
fall asleep as automobile driver [2]	1.2
fall asleep as automobile passenger [1]	15.7

Symptom	%
fall asleep as automobile passenger [2]	16.2
fall asleep at school or church [1]	3.2
fall asleep at school or church [2]	1.5
fall asleep at work [1]	1.3
fall asleep at work [2]	0.6
fall asleep reading or watching TV [1]	27.3
fall asleep reading or watching TV [2]	20.1
fall asleep: after a meal [1]	11.7
fall asleep: after a meal [2]	11.1

Fernandez & Sheffield (1996)
n = 91
Diagnostic Criteria:
Gender: 91/0
Age: 39.3 (12.8)
Race:

Population Setting: headache study
volunteers
Nationality: Australia
Other Sample Characteristics:
Method of Reporting: self-report
Timeframe: 12 months

Symptom	%
combined headache	16.5
migraine headache	19.8

Symptom	%
other headache	41.8
tension headache	22.0

Fernandez & Sheffield (1996)
n = 170
Diagnostic Criteria:
Gender: 0/170
Age: 35.1 (11.7)
Race:

Population Setting: headache study
volunteers
Nationality: Australia
Other Sample Characteristics:

Method of Reporting: self-report   Timeframe: 12 months

Symptom	%
combined headache	26.5
migraine headache	19.4

Symptom	%
other headache	28.8
tension headache	25.3

Fernandez & Sheffield (1996)
n = 261
Diagnostic Criteria:
Gender: 91/170
Age: 36.6 (12.3)
Race:

Population Setting: headache study
volunteers
Nationality: Australia
Other Sample Characteristics:
Method of Reporting: self-report
Timeframe: 12 months

Symptom	%
combined headache	22
migraine headache	19

Symptom	%
other headache	33
tension headache	24

Lavie (1981)
n = 1502
Diagnostic Criteria:
Gender: 1262/240
Age:
Race:
Population Setting: industrial workers

Nationality: Israel
Other Sample Characteristics: [1]while
falling asleep, [2]while sleeping,
[3]awakening
Method of Reporting: structured
interview
Timeframe: 12 months

Symptom	%
difficulties breathing and suffocating [3]	3.0
difficulty breathing and suffocation [1]	5.8
disorientation [1]	1.6
disorientation [3]	1.0
excessive leg movements [2]	9.6
excessive movements in sleep [2]	33.2
feelings of worry and tension [1]	12.0
headaches [1]	7.2
headaches [3]	5.5
midsleep awakening [3]	17

Symptom	%
pain in different parts of the body [1]	7.5
pain in different parts of the body [3]	4.7
paralysis of the legs [1]	0.7
paralysis of the legs [3]	0.5
sleep walking [2]	0.4
snoring [2]	18.5
sweating and feeling hot [1]	7.5
sweating and feeling hot [3]	4.3

talking in one's sleep [2]	3.6

worries and tension [3]	1.4

Lavie (1981)
n = 1262
Diagnostic Criteria:
Gender: 1262/0
Age:
Race:

Population Setting: industrial workers
Nationality: Israel
Other Sample Characteristics:
Method of Reporting: structured interview
Timeframe: 12 months

Symptom	%
difficulties falling asleep	6.6
difficulties falling asleep and midsleep awakenings	2.7
EDS and difficulties falling asleep and midsleep awakening	3.1

Symptom	%
excessive daytime somnolence	5.0
midsleep awakening	10.8

Lavie (1981)
n = 240
Diagnostic Criteria:
Gender: 0/240
Age:
Race:

Population Setting: industrial workers
Nationality: Israel
Other Sample Characteristics:
Method of Reporting: structured interview
Timeframe: 12 months

Symptom	%
difficulties falling asleep	12.1
difficulties falling asleep and midsleep awakenings	7.1
EDS and difficulties falling asleep and midsleep awakenings	2.1

Symptom	%
excessive daytime somnolence	4.6
midsleep awakenings	12.1

Droller & Pemberton (1953)
n = 476
Diagnostic Criteria:
Gender: [1]192/0, [2]0/284
Age: [1]67+, [2]62+
Race:

Population Setting: industrial workers
Nationality: Israel
Other Sample Characteristics:
Method of Reporting: medical exam
Timeframe:

Symptom	%
vertigo [1]	27.6

vertigo [2]	53.9

Hannay (1978)
n = 1,344
Diagnostic Criteria:
Gender:
Age:
Race:

Population Setting: community
Nationality: UK
Other Sample Characteristics:
Method of Reporting: interview
Timeframe: 2 weeks

Symptom	%
absence of periods and probably not pregnant	0.1
absence of periods and probably pregnant	0.4
ankle swelling in both ankles	4.6
ankle swelling in both ankles and varicose veins	1.8
attacks of breathlessness when lying down	0.5
attacks of breathlessness when lying down and sudden attacks of breathlessness when lying down at night	0.1
attacks of palpitations or breathlessness	7.5
attacks of palpitations when heart beats fast for no apparent reason	4.5
attacks of palpitations when heart beats fast for no apparent reason and attacks of breathlessness when lying down	0.2
attacks of palpitations when heart beats fast for no apparent reason and sudden attacks of breathlessness when lying down at night	0.4

Symptom	%
attacks of palpitations when heart beats fast for no apparent reason, attacks of breathlessness when lying down, and sudden attacks of breathlessness when lying down at night	0.8
attacks of shortness of breath with wheezing	1.0
bleeding between periods, or post menopausal	0.1
boils or other skin trouble	1.7
bunions, corns, or callosites	0.1
bunions, corns, or callosites	14.3
bunions, corns, or callosites, and flat feet or other	0.3
bunions, corns, or callosites, and ingrown toenails	0.4
bunions, corns, or callosites, ingrown toenails, and flat feet or other	0.1
burn	1.1
change in weight	8.7
change of appetite	7.9
chest sounding wheezy or whistling	3.9

chest sounding wheezy or whistling and attacks of shortness of breath with wheezing	2.5
chest sounding wheezy or whistling and coughing up blood which had not been swallowed	0.1
chest sounding wheezy or whistling, attacks of shortness of breath with wheezing, and coughing up blood which had not been swallowed	0.1
comes on only when walking and goes in 10 minutes or less if stands still	1.3
comes on when standing still or sitting and comes on when walking and goes in 10 minutes or less if stand still	0.2
comes on when standing still or walking	1.0
constipation	4.2
convulsions or fits	0.4
cough now or during the past two weeks	0.2
cough now or during the past two weeks	15.9
cough now or during the past two weeks and usually cough first on getting up	5.8
cough up blood which had not been swallowed	0.1
dandruff	4.0
diarrhea	1.7
difficulty in eating because of mouth or gums	1.9

difficulty in eating because of mouth or gums and difficulty in swallowing because of trouble in throat (or esophagus)	0.1
difficulty in hearing	0.1
difficulty in hearing	8.2
difficulty in hearing and ringing or buzzing in ears	0.6
difficulty in seeing	6.4
difficulty in seeing and loss of sight in one or both eyes	0.1
difficulty in swallowing because of trouble in throat (or esophagus)	0.9
difficulty or discomfort in passing water	2.2
discharge and irritation in private parts	0.7
discharge in private parts	1.6
discomfort such as pain or burning while passing water	1.2
facial pain, loss of speech or balance	2.6
feeling more irritable and jumpy than usual	1.3
feeling more thirsty than usual or cold apart from the weather	5.7
fever	2.5
fever and unusual flushing	0.1
fever and unusual sweating	0.7
fever and unusual sweating and flushing	0.1
flat feet or other	4.5
gain in weight	5.4
gain of appetite or feeling hungry	2.7
generally run down	1.6
having to run to toilet	0.4

having to run to toilet and water leaks when straining, coughing, or laughing	1.3
having to stop for breath when walking at own pace on level ground"	2.5
headaches	0.1
headaches	12.9
headaches and spells of dizziness or vertigo	2.0
headaches, and feeling more irritable and jumpy than usual	1.0
headaches, spells of dizziness or vertigo, and feeling more irritable and jumpy than usual	1.2
heartburn	6.3
heartburn and indigestion	2.2
heartburn or indigestion	14.7
hoarseness or loss of voice	3.6
hoarseness or loss of voice and other trouble with throat or voice	0.1
indigestion	6.3
ingrown toenails	1.4
ingrown toenails and flat feet or other	0.1
irregularity of periods	2.5
irritation in private parts	0.7
loss of ability to balance on feet	1.2
loss of appetite	5.2
loss of consciousness or blackouts	1.2
loss of feeling, tingling, or numbness in lower limbs	2.4
loss of feeling, tingling, or numbness in upper and lower limbs	1.5
loss of feeling, tingling, or numbness in upper limbs	3.8
loss of hair	1.0

loss of power in lower limbs	0.7
loss of power in upper and lower limbs	0.5
loss of power in upper limbs	0.8
loss of power of speech	0.4
loss of power of speech and loss of ability to balance on feet	0.1
loss of sight in one or both eyes	1.2
loss of weight	3.3
low back pain	5.4
low back pain and pain elsewhere in spine	0.2
low back pain and pain in large bones	0.3
low back pain, pain elsewhere in spine, and pain in large bones	0.4
lumps in breast	0.1
lumps or swollen glands (other than in breasts)	4.2
more cold apart from the weather	1.4
more thirsty than usual	3.6
more thirsty than usual and more cold apart from the weather	0.7
more tired than usual	16.1
more tired than usual	0.2
more tired than usual and generally run down	5.0
morning sickness and other with pregnancy	0.1
morning sickness with pregnancy	0.1
morning sickness. pain or bleeding, and other with pregnancy	0.1
morning stiffness in joints	0.7

nausea or feeling like vomiting	3.3
nose bleeds	0.6
other	0.2
other discoloration such as bruising	0.5
other minor injury or accident such as a fall with bruising	7.7
other pain in calf or either leg	6.0
other pain or discomfort in chest	3.8
other serious injury or accident such as fall with broken bone	0.4
other trouble with throat or voice	0.2
pain elsewhere in spine	2.5
pain elsewhere in spine and pain in large bones	0.6
pain in abdomen or tummy	5.1
pain in abdomen or tummy and constipation	0.7
pain in abdomen or tummy and diarrhea	0.7
pain in abdomen or tummy and diarrhea and constipation	0.1
pain in calf of either leg	8.5
pain in face for no apparent reason	0.7
pain in face for no apparent reason, loss of power of speech, and loss of ability to balance on feet	0.1
pain in large bones	5.0
pain in private parts	0.2
pain on defecation	1.1
pain on defecation and red blood on stool or paper	0.4

pain or bleeding with pregnancy	0.1
pain or bleeding with pregnancy and other	0.1
pain or discomfort in chest which may go to arm comes on walking and goes in 10 minutes or less if stop or slow down	1.9
pain or swelling in private parts or front passage	0.4
pain with last period	1.5
pain with last period and unusually heavy	0.3
pain, irritation, or watering of eyes	6.3
pain, irritation, or watering of eyes and difficulty in seeing	1.0
pain, irritation, or watering of eyes and loss of sight in one or both eyes	0.2
pain, irritation, or wax in ears	3.8
pain, irritation, or wax in ears and difficulty in hearing	1.0
pain, irritation, or wax in ears, and ringing and buzzing in ears	0.4
pain, irritation, or wax in ears, difficulty in hearing, and ringing or buzzing in ears	0.5
pain, swelling, tenderness, and redness in small joints of hands or feet and morning stiffness of joints	0.3
pain, swelling, tenderness, and redness in small joints of hands or feet, and in large joints, and morning stiffness in joints	0.9
pain, swelling, tenderness, or redness in large joints	4.7

pain, swelling, tenderness, or redness in large joints, and morning stiffness in joints	0.3
pain, swelling, tenderness, or redness in small joints of hands or feet	3.6
pain, swelling, tenderness, or redness in small joints of hands or feet, and in large joints	0.7
paler than usual skin or whites of eyes	0.9
passing water more difficult than usual	0.7
passing water more difficult than usual or discomfort such as pain or burning while passing water	0.2
passing water more frequently at night	1.8
passing water more frequently during the day	1.6
passing water more frequently during the day and at night	2.2
passing water more often than usual	5.6
rash or irritation	12.4
rash or irritation and boils or other skin trouble	0.1
rash or irritation and sores or ulcers on skin	0.1
rash or irritations	0.1
red blood on stool or paper	0.8
reddish/brown discoloration about water	0.3
retching without bringing up food	1.1
ringing or buzzing in ears	1.3
severe pain across front of chest which lasts for half an hour or more	1.3

severe pain across front of chest which lasts for half an hour or more and other pain or discomfort in chest	0.1
shortness of breath	19.3
shortness of breath when	0.1
sore throat	6.6
sore throat and hoarseness or loss of voice	0.9
sores or ulcers on skin	0.8
spells of dizziness or vertigo	4.9
spells of dizziness or vertigo and feeling more irritable and jumpy than usual	0.3
sputum now or during the past two weeks	0.1
sputum now or during the past two weeks	8.7
sputum now or during the past two weeks and usually first thing on getting up	4.5
strong smell about water	0.7
stuffy or runny nose or catarrh at back of nose	0.2
stuffy or runny nose, or catarrh at back of nose	26.4
stuffy or runny nose, or catarrh at back of nose and nose bleeds	0.1
sudden attacks of breathlessness when lying down at night	0.9
superfluous hair	0.0
swelling in private parts	0.1
swellings such as a rupture	0.4
trouble with teeth	7.8
trouble with teeth and difficulty in eating because of mouth or gums	0.4

trouble with water coming too quickly	2.4
unusual color or smell about water	1.3
unusual flushing	1.6
unusual sweating	2.2
unusual sweating and flushing	0.5
unusually heavy last period	0.7
usually cough first thing on getting up	0.2
usually cough first upon getting up	6.3
usually sputum first thing on getting up	0.1
usually sputum first thing on getting up	6.5

varicose veins	0.2
varicose veins	9.3
vomiting up blood which had not been swallowed	0.1
vomiting up food or drink	4.4
water leaks when straining, coughing, or laughing	0.7
when hurrying on level ground or walking up slight hill	12.4
when sitting quietly	1.7
when walking with people of own age on level ground	1.3
when washing or dressing	1.5
yellower than usual skin or whites of eyes	0.2

Enright, et al. (1994)
n = 1643
Diagnostic Criteria:
Gender: 0/1643
Age: 65+
Race:
Population Setting: community

Nationality: US
Other Sample Characteristics: non-smokers
Method of Reporting: structured interview
Timeframe:

Symptom	%
cough > 3 months	7.4
cough day and night	9.1
frequent cough	8.2
frequent phlegm	8.0
grade 3 dyspnea	10.0

Symptom	%
phlegm > 3 months	7.9
phlegm day and night	7.4
wheeze and dyspnea	6.9
wheeze day and night	4.1

Enright, et al. (1994)
n = 716
Diagnostic Criteria:
Gender: 716/0
Age: 65+
Race:
Population Setting: community

Nationality: US
Other Sample Characteristics: non-smokers
Method of Reporting: structured interview
Timeframe:

Symptom	%
cough > 3 months	5.7
cough day and night	5.7
dyspnea grade 3	6.4
frequent cough	6.1
frequent phlegm	12.5

Symptom	%
phlegm > 3 months	11.5
phlegm day and night	11.4
wheeze and dyspnea	6.0
wheeze day and night	3.2

Enright, et al. (1994)
n = 875
Diagnostic Criteria:
Gender: 0/875
Age: 65+
Race:
Population Setting: community

Nationality: US
Other Sample Characteristics: former
smokers
Method of Reporting: structured
interview
Timeframe:

Symptom	%
cough > 3 months	7.5
cough day and night	8.6
dyspnea grade 3	12.5
frequent cough	8.6
frequent phlegm	10.3

Symptom	%
phlegm > 3 months	9.9
phlegm day and night	8.6
wheeze and dyspnea	9.8
wheeze day and night	4.5

Enright, et al. (1994)
n = 1272
Diagnostic Criteria:
Gender: 1272/0
Age: 65+
Race:
Population Setting: community

Nationality: US
Other Sample Characteristics: former
smokers
Method of Reporting: structured
interview
Timeframe:

Symptom	%
cough > 3 months	7.6
cough day and night	8.1
dyspnea grade 3	9.6
frequent cough	7.6
frequent phlegm	15.4

Symptom	%
phlegm > 3 months	16.0
phlegm day and night	14.5
wheeze and dyspnea	7.2
wheeze day and night	5.7

Enright, et al. (1994)
n = 382
Diagnostic Criteria:

Gender: 0/382
Age: 65+
Race:

Population Setting: community
Nationality: US
Other Sample Characteristics: current
smokers

Method of Reporting: structured
interview
Timeframe:

Symptom	%
cough > 3 months	22.8
cough day and night	24.3
dyspnea grade 3	11.5
frequent cough	25.1
frequent phlegm	27.7

Symptom	%
phlegm > 3 months	23.8
phlegm day and night	25.1
wheeze and dyspnea	10.2
wheeze day and night	10.7

Enright, et al. (1994)
n = 231
Diagnostic Criteria:
Gender: 231/0
Age: 65+
Race:
Population Setting: community

Nationality: US
Other Sample Characteristics: current
smokers
Method of Reporting: structured
interview
Timeframe:

Symptom	%
cough > 3 months	9.2
cough day and night	10.5
dyspnea grade 3	10.1
frequent cough	10
frequent phlegm	13.8

Symptom	%
phlegm > 3 months	13.1
phlegm day and night	12.4
wheeze and dyspnea	7.7
wheeze day and night	5.6

Katona, et al. (1997)
n = 700
Diagnostic Criteria:
Gender: 253/447
Age: 65+
Race:

Population Setting: community
Nationality: UK
Other Sample Characteristics:
Method of Reporting: semi-structured
interview
Timeframe:

Symptom	%
difficulty falling asleep	21
difficulty with light housework	14
does not get out as often as needs to	21

Symptom	%
embarrassed by memory problems	13
faintness on rapid rising	11
feeling dizzy	21
feeling weak	12

forgets where put things	26
health getting worse	9
health limiting mobility	24
health limiting other activities	17
health limiting socializing	7
health problems interfering with desired activity	50

interrupted sleep	33
making effort to remember things	14
not eating well	7
subjective memory difficulty	34

Newland, et al. (1978)
n = 46
Diagnostic Criteria:
Gender: 46/0
Age: 18-20
Race:

Population Setting: community
Nationality: UK
Other Sample Characteristics:
Method of Reporting: postal survey
Timeframe: 1 year

Symptom	%
blind areas before headache	2
changes in mood before headache	14
headache	87
pins and needles before headache	0

Symptom	%
sickness before headache	7
watery eyes before headache	6
zigzag flashes before headache	1

Newland, et al. (1978)
n = 233
Diagnostic Criteria:
Gender: 233/0
Age: 21-34
Race:

Population Setting: community
Nationality: UK
Other Sample Characteristics:
Method of Reporting: postal survey
Timeframe: 1 year

Symptom	%
blind areas before headache	8
changes in mood before headache	47
headache	88
pins and needles before headache	7

Symptom	%
sickness before headache	36
watery eyes before headache	38
zigzag flashes before headache	10

Newland, et al. (1978)
n = 320
Diagnostic Criteria:
Gender: 320/0
Age: 35-54
Race:

Population Setting: community
Nationality: UK
Other Sample Characteristics:
Method of Reporting: postal survey
Timeframe: 1 year

Symptom	%
blind areas before headache	21.0
changes in mood before headache	53.0
headache	80.3
pins and needles before headache	8.0

Symptom	%
sickness before headache	64.0
watery eyes before headache	45.0
zigzag flashes before headache	21.0

Newland, et al. (1978)
n = 284
Diagnostic Criteria:
Gender: 284/0
Age: 55-74
Race:

Population Setting: community
Nationality: UK
Other Sample Characteristics:
Method of Reporting: postal survey
Timeframe: 1 year

Symptom	%
blind areas before headache	16
changes in mood before headache	35
headache	56
pins and needles before headache	8

Symptom	%
sickness before headache	20
watery eyes before headache	32
zigzag flashes before headache	15

Newland, et al. (1978)
n = 55
Diagnostic Criteria:
Gender: 55/0
Age: 75+
Race:

Population Setting: community
Nationality: UK
Other Sample Characteristics:
Method of Reporting: postal survey
Timeframe: 1 year

Symptom	%
blind areas before headache	2.0
changes in mood before headache	3.0
headache	45.5
pins and needles before headache	1.0

Symptom	%
sickness before headache	3.0
watery eyes before headache	8.0
zigzag flashes before headache	1.0

Newland, et al. (1978)
n = 63
Diagnostic Criteria:
Gender: 0/63
Age: 18-20
Race:

Population Setting: community
Nationality: UK
Other Sample Characteristics:
Method of Reporting: postal survey
Timeframe: 1 year

Symptom	%
blind areas before headache	2.0
changes in mood before headache	17
headache	93.7
pins and needles before headache	0.0

Symptom	%
sickness before headache	11.0
watery eyes before headache	14.0
zigzag flashes before headache	3.0

Newland, et al. (1978)
n = 276
Diagnostic Criteria:
Gender: 0/276
Age: 21-34
Race:

Population Setting: community
Nationality: UK
Other Sample Characteristics:
Method of Reporting: postal survey
Timeframe: 1 year

Symptom	%
blind areas before headache	13.0
changes in mood before headache	86.0
headache	96.7
pins and needles before headache	14.0

Symptom	%
sickness before headache	87.0
watery eyes before headache	84.0
zigzag flashes before headache	23.0

Newland, et al. (1978)
n = 314
Diagnostic Criteria:
Gender: 0/314
Age: 35-54
Race:

Population Setting: community
Nationality: UK
Other Sample Characteristics:
Method of Reporting: postal survey
Timeframe: 1 year

Symptom	%
blind areas before headache	24.0
changes in mood before headache	93.0
headache	91.1
pins and needles before headache	13.0

Symptom	%
sickness before headache	96.0
watery eyes before headache	56.0
zigzag flashes before headache	24.0

Newland, et al. (1978)
n = 363
Diagnostic Criteria:
Gender: 0/363
Age: 55-74
Race:

Population Setting: community
Nationality: UK
Other Sample Characteristics:
Method of Reporting: postal survey
Timeframe: 1 year

Symptom	%
blind areas before headache	15
changes in mood before headache	63
headache	68
pins and needles before headache	24

Symptom	%
sickness before headache	63
watery eyes before headache	58
zigzag flashes before headache	38

Newland, et al. (1978)
n = 110
Diagnostic Criteria:
Gender: 0/110
Age: 75+
Race:

Population Setting: community
Nationality: UK
Other Sample Characteristics:
Method of Reporting: postal survey
Timeframe: 1 year

Symptom	%
changes in mood before headache	6.0
headache	52.7
pins and needles before headache	2.0
blind areas before headache	6.0

Symptom	%
sickness before headache	9.0
watery eyes before headache	18.0
zigzag flashes before headache	7.0

Schaughency, et al. (1994)
n = 943
Diagnostic Criteria:
Gender: 483/460
Age: 15
Race:

Population Setting: community
Nationality: New Zealand
Other Sample Characteristics:
Method of Reporting: self-report
Timeframe: current

Symptom	%
hard time to finish something enjoy	7.9
hard to sit still	7.3
hard to sit through something	9.7
has hard time doing schoolwork with noises/ other things going on	19.8
has trouble paying attention when people are talking	3.1
often start on schoolwork and not finish	15.3
run around a lot inside home or school when not supposed to	5.3

Symptom	%
rush into doing things without thinking what may happen	17.3
teacher has to remind what to do again and again	3.3
teacher says not keeping mind on work	7.5
trouble organizing schoolwork	7.7
trouble waiting turn or push ahead in line	3.6

Schaughency, et al. (1994)
n = 483
Diagnostic Criteria:
Gender: 483/0
Age: 15
Race:

Population Setting: community
Nationality: New Zealand
Other Sample Characteristics:
Method of Reporting: self-report
Timeframe: current

Symptom	%
hard time to finish something enjoy	7.3
hard to sit still	7.0
hard to sit through something	8.9
has hard time doing schoolwork with noises/ other things going on	21.3
has trouble paying attention when people are talking	2.7
often start on schoolwork and not finish	13.7
run around a lot inside home or school when not supposed to	6.0

Symptom	%
rush into doing things without thinking what may happen	19.5
teacher has to remind what to do again and again	2.5
teacher says not keeping mind on work	6.0
trouble organizing schoolwork	7.9
trouble waiting turn or push ahead in line	3.9

Schaughency, et al. (1994)
n = 460
Diagnostic Criteria:
Gender: 0/460
Age: 15
Race:

Population Setting: community
Nationality: New Zealand
Other Sample Characteristics:
Method of Reporting: self-report
Timeframe: current

Symptom	%
hard time to finish something enjoy	8.5
hard to sit still	7.6
hard to sit through something	10.4
has hard time doing schoolwork with noises/other things going on	18.3
has trouble paying attention when people are talking	3.7
often start on schoolwork and not finish	17.2
run around a lot inside home or school when not supposed to	4.6

Symptom	%
rush into doing things without thinking what may happen	15.0
teacher has to remind what to do again and again	4.1
teacher says not keeping mind on work	9.1
trouble organizing schoolwork	7.6
trouble waiting turn or push ahead in line	3.3

Schaughency, et al. (1994)
n = 397
Diagnostic Criteria:
Gender: 397/0
Age: 18
Race:

Population Setting: community
Nationality: New Zealand
Other Sample Characteristics:
Method of Reporting: other-report
Timeframe: current

Symptom	%
impairment	7.2
impulsivity	45.7

Symptom	%
inattention	36.9

Schaughency, et al. (1994)
n = 394
Diagnostic Criteria:
Gender: 0/394
Age: 18
Race:

Population Setting: community
Nationality: New Zealand
Other Sample Characteristics:
Method of Reporting: other-report
Timeframe: current

Symptom	%
impairment	4.3
impulsivity	41.6

Symptom	%
inattention	33.3

Kanbayashi, et al. (1994)
n = 1,022
Diagnostic Criteria:
Gender: 492/509
Age: 4-12
Race:

Population Setting: public school
Nationality: Japan
Other Sample Characteristics:
Method of Reporting: teacher report
Timeframe: current

Symptom	%
blurts out answers before the question is completed	20.3
difficulty following through on instructions from others	6.5
difficulty playing quietly	12.2
difficulty sustaining attention in tasks or play	17.9
does not seem to listen to what is being said	27.2

Symptom	%
fidgets with hand or feet or squirms in seat	14.9
has difficulty awaiting turn	5.8
has difficulty remaining seated	14.5
interrupts or intrudes on others	11.0
is easily distracted	35.7

often engages in dangerous activities without considering the consequences	17.1
often loses things necessary for tests or activities	25.8
often talks excessively	29.6

shifts from one uncompleted activity to another	33.6

Kanbayashi, et al. (1994)
n = 198
Diagnostic Criteria:
Gender: 198/0
Age: 4-6
Race:

Population Setting: public school
Nationality: Japan
Other Sample Characteristics:
Method of Reporting: teacher report
Timeframe: current

Symptom	%
blurts out answers before the question is completed	23.2
difficulty following through on instructions from others	9.1
difficulty playing quietly	19.7
difficulty sustaining attention in tasks or play	21.2
does not seem to listen to what is being said	29.8
fidgets with hand or feet or squirms in seat	18.2
has difficulty awaiting turn	10.6
has difficulty remaining seated	26.3

Symptom	%
interrupts or intrudes on others	17.7
is easily distracted	43.4
often engages in dangerous activities without considering the consequences	33.8
often loses things necessary for tasks or activities	22.7
often talks excessively	31.3
shifts from one uncompleted activity to another	35.9

Kanbayashi, et al. (1994)
n = 215
Diagnostic Criteria:
Gender: 0/215
Age: 4-6
Race:

Population Setting: public school
Nationality: Japan
Other Sample Characteristics:
Method of Reporting: teacher report
Timeframe: current

Symptom	%
blurts out answers before the question is completed	26.5
difficulty following through on instructions from others	4.7
difficulty playing quietly	11.1
difficulty sustaining attention in tasks or play	18.6
does not seem to listen to what is being said	24.2
fidgets with hand or feet or squirms in seat	14.4
has difficulty awaiting turn	7.0
has difficulty remaining seated	14.4

Symptom	%
interrupts or intrudes on others	16.6
is easily distracted	44.2
often engages in dangerous activities without considering the consequences	21.4
often loses things necessary for tests or activities	23.7
often talks excessively	39.5
shifts from one uncompleted activity to another	44.7

Kanbayashi, et al. (1994)
n = 153
Diagnostic Criteria:
Gender: 153/0
Age: 7-9
Race:

Population Setting: public school
Nationality: Japan
Other Sample Characteristics:
Method of Reporting: teacher report
Timeframe: current

Symptom	%
blurts out answers before the question is completed	25.5
difficulty following through on instructions from others	11.8
difficulty playing quietly	18.3
difficulty sustaining attention in tasks or play	26.8
does not seem to listen to what is being said	37.3
fidgets with hand or feet or squirms in seat	26.8
has difficulty awaiting turn	8.5

Symptom	%
has difficulty remaining seated	21.6
interrupts or intrudes on others	11.1
is easily distracted	47.7
often engages in dangerous activities without considering the consequences	19.6
often loses things necessary for tests or activities	41.2
often talks excessively	32.7

	%
shifts from one uncompleted activity to another	36.0

Kanbayashi, et al. (1994)
n = 121
Diagnostic Criteria:
Gender: 0/121
Age: 7-9
Race:

Population Setting: public school
Nationality: Japan
Other Sample Characteristics:
Method of Reporting: teacher report
Timeframe: current

Symptom	%
blurts out answers before the question is completed	12.4
blurts out answers before the question is completed	4.1
difficulty playing quietly	8.3
difficulty sustaining attention in tasks or play	14.1
does not seem to listen to what is being said	24
fidgets with hand or feet or squirms in seat	7.4
has difficulty awaiting turn	1.7
has difficulty remaining seated	9.1

Symptom	%
interrupts or intrudes on others	3.3
is easily distracted	28.1
often engages in dangerous activities without considering the consequences	9.9
often loses things necessary for tests or activities	24.8
often talks excessively	31.4
shifts from one uncompleted activity to another	31.4

Kanbayashi, et al. (1994)
n = 141
Diagnostic Criteria:
Gender: 141/0
Age: 10-12
Race:

Population Setting: public school
Nationality: Japan
Other Sample Characteristics:
Method of Reporting: teacher report
Timeframe: current

Symptom	%
blurts out answers before question is completed	24.1
difficulty following through on instructions from others	6.4
difficulty playing quietly	10.6

Symptom	%
difficulty sustaining attention in tasks or play	19.2
does not seem to listen to what is being said	34.0

fidgets with hand or feet or squirms in seat	15.6
has difficulty awaiting turn	4.3
has difficulty remaining seated	10.6
interrupts or intrudes on others	7.1
is easily distracted	34.0

often engages in dangerous activities without considering the consequences	8.5
often loses things necessary for tests or activities	34.8
often talks excessively	23.4
shifts from one uncompleted activity to another	36.2

Kanbayashi, et al. (1994)
n = 173
Diagnostic Criteria:
Gender: 0/173
Age: 10-12
Race:

Population Setting: public school
Nationality: Japan
Other Sample Characteristics:
Method of Reporting: teacher report
Timeframe: current

Symptom	%
blurts out answers before question is completed	9.8
difficulty following through on instructions from others	3.5
difficulty playing quietly	5.2
difficulty sustaining attention in tasks or play	9.3
does not seem to listen to what is being said	19.1
fidgets with hand or feet or squirms in seat	7.5
has difficulty awaiting turn	1.2
has difficulty remaining seated	3.5

Symptom	%
interrupts or intrudes on others	6.4
is easily distracted	16.8
often engages in dangerous activities without considering the consequences	4.6
often loses things necessary for tests or activities	15.0
often talks excessively	20.2
shifts from one uncompleted activity to another	19.1

Kanbayashi, et al. (1994)
n = 944
Diagnostic Criteria:
Gender: 514/508
Age: 4-12
Race:

Population Setting: public school
Nationality: Japan
Other Sample Characteristics:
Method of Reporting: teacher rating
Timeframe: current

Symptom	%
inattentiveness	5.7
hyperactive-ness	2.0
impulsiveness	1.3

Symptom	%
disobedience	0.8
school refusal	0.1

Jebbink, et al. (1994)
n = 12
Diagnostic Criteria:
Gender: 7/5
Age: 46.3 (3.7)
Race:

Population Setting: community
Nationality: Netherlands
Other Sample Characteristics: post-
prandial
Method of Reporting: self-report
Timeframe: 1 week

Symptom	%
fullness, early satiety, and bloating post pradially	0
nausea and vomiting	42

Hinds, et al. (1990)
n = 78
Diagnostic Criteria:
Gender: 17/61
Age: 42.0 (22-64)
Race:

Population Setting: hospital workers
Nationality: Netherlands
Other Sample Characteristics:
Method of Reporting: postal survey
Timeframe: 1 week

Symptom	%
constipation	9
depression	3
dysphagia	13
fecal incontinence	4

Symptom	%
heartburn	33
hemorrhoids	19
peptic ulcer	9
urinary dysfunction	5

Carlson & Kashani. (1988)
n = 150
Diagnostic Criteria:
Gender: 75/75
Age: 14-16
Race:
Population Setting: community

Nationality: US
Other Sample Characteristics:
Method of Reporting: interview of
parent and adolescent, DICA-
P/DICA)
Timeframe: lifetime

Symptom	%
during that "high" period, did you feel your thoughts were coming too fast	8.0
during that high period, did you do things you wished you hadn't	6.6
during that high period, did you have a hard time paying attention	9.3
during that high period, did you sleep a lot less w/out feeling tired	8.7
during that high period, did you talk faster or a lot more than usual	10.0
during that high period, did you think you had a special disability	6.6

Symptom	%
during that high period, were you much more active than usual	4.7
have you ever gone through a period when you become unusually excited	4.0
have you ever gone through a period when you couldn't sleep at night because of so much energy	8.0
have you ever gone through a time when your mood went up and down quickly	10.0

Sloane, Blazer, George (1989)
$\underline{n}$ = 1,620
Diagnostic Criteria:
Gender:
Age: [1]60-64; [2]65-69; [3]70-74; [4]75-79; [5]80-84; [6]85+
Race:
Population Setting: community

Nationality: US
Other Sample Characteristics:
severity criteria: resulting in a physician visit, in taking a medication more than once, or interfering with activities "a lot"
Method of Reporting: self-report
Timeframe: 1 year

Symptom	%
dizziness[1]	17.8
dizziness[2]	15.6
dizziness[3]	18.7

Symptom	%
dizziness[4]	20.1
dizziness[5]	23.8
dizziness[6]	21.3

Bowling (1990)
$\underline{n}$ = 662
Diagnostic Criteria:
Gender: 126/536
Age: 85+
Race:

Population Setting: community
Nationality: UK
Other Sample Characteristics:
Method of Reporting: self-report
Timeframe: current

Symptom	%
abdominal pain	29

Symptom	%
aches/pains/stiff	84

muscles/joints	
alternate constipation/loose	11
chest pain/heart trouble	34
constipation	39
depressed/suicidal thoughts	15
feelings of anxiety	29
forgetfulness	44

giddiness	50
headache	28
loss of appetite	30
nerves/stress depression	62
piles	18
poor perceived health and feelings of poor self worth	49
sleeplessness	61
urinary incontinence	40

Judd, Rapaport, Paulus, et al. (1994)
$n = 9,160$
Diagnostic Criteria:
Gender: 4,195/4,965
Age: 18+
Race: 5111/2125/1392/238/82/211

Population Setting: community
Nationality: US
Other Sample Characteristics:
Method of Reporting: structured interview
Timeframe: 1 month

Symptom	%
a lot more trouble concentrating	9
increased appetite; gained as much as two pounds per week	9.5
less interest in sex than usual	9.5
sleeping too much	8.7

Symptom	%
tired out all the time	22.8
trouble falling asleep, staying asleep, waking up early	33.7

Garrison, Schluchter, Schoenbach, et al. (1989)
$n = 677$
Diagnostic Criteria:
Gender:
Age: 11-17
Race: 542/135/0/0/0/0

Population Setting: public junior high school students
Nationality: US
Other Sample Characteristics:
Method of Reporting: self report
Timeframe: 1 week

Symptom	%
bothered by things	59
could not get going	61
could not shake blues	45
doesn't feel like eating	41
enjoyed life	58
everything was an effort	81
felt depressed	56
felt fearful	34

Symptom	%
felt lonely	47
felt people disliked me	51
felt sad	53
had crying spells	22
hopeful about the future	71
just as good as others	65
life had been a failure	29
people were unfriendly	48

sleep was restless	47
talked less than usual	58
trouble keeping mind on	78

things	
was happy	64

Kivela, Nissinen, Tuomilehto, et al. (1986)
n = 321
Diagnostic Criteria:
Gender: 321/0
Age: 65-84
Race:

Population Setting: community
Nationality: Finland
Other Sample Characteristics: [1]East Residence; [2]South West Residence
Method of Reporting: self report
Timeframe: 2 weeks

Symptom	%
apathy and feebleness[1]	54
apathy and feebleness[2]	46
chest pain[1]	52
chest pain[2]	41
constipation[1]	35
constipation[2]	30
diarrhea[1]	20
diarrhea[2]	20
dizziness[1]	53
dizziness[2]	51
dry mouth[1]	42
dry mouth[2]	38
dypsnea on exertion[1]	70
dypsnea on exertion[2]	58
dyspnea at rest[1]	33
dyspnea at rest[2]	24
falling[1]	10
falling[2]	7
fatigue and weakness[1]	65
fatigue and weakness[2]	54
frequent sweating[1]	27
frequent sweating[2]	28
frequent thirst[1]	18
frequent thirst[2]	19
headache[1]	50
headache[2]	0
hearing disturbances[1]	51
hearing disturbances[2]	45
itching skin[1]	34
itching skin[2]	26
joint pain[1]	60

Symptom	%
joint pain[2]	47
loss of appetite[1]	24
loss of appetite[2]	18
memory difficulties[1]	70
memory difficulties[2]	65
muscle pain[1]	62
muscle pain[2]	41
nausea[1]	36
nausea[2]	24
neck pain[1]	68
neck pain[2]	55
pain on urinating[1]	46
pain on urinating[2]	10
palpitations[1]	47
palpitations[2]	43
restlessness[1]	35
restlessness[2]	26
sight disturbances[1]	33
sight disturbances[2]	20
stomach pain[1]	45
stomach pain[2]	28
tremor[1]	30
tremor[2]	30
urinary frequency[1]	46
urinary frequency[2]	50
urinary incontinence[1]	17
urinary incontinence[2]	18
vomiting[1]	11
vomiting[2]	8

Kivela & Pahkela (1988)
$\underline{n} = 330$
Diagnostic Criteria:
Gender: [1]138/[2]192
Age: [1]69.7 (7.0); [2]71.1 (7.3)
Race:

Population Setting: community
Nationality: Finland
Other Sample Characteristics:
Method of Reporting: physician's
assessment
Timeframe: current

Symptom	%
anorexia[1]	1
anorexia[2]	6
auditory hallucinations[1]	0
auditory hallucinations[2]	0
concentration loss[1]	4
concentration loss[2]	6
constipation[1]	5
constipation[2]	11
crying spells[1]	2
crying spells[2]	1
crying spells[1]	1
crying spells[2]	1
decreased life satisfaction[1]	1
decreased life satisfaction[2]	0
delusions of unforgivable behavior[1]	1
delusions of unforgivable behavior[2]	2
delusions of uselessness[1]	0
delusions of uselessness[2]	0
depressed mood[1]	8
depressed mood[2]	0
emptiness[1]	0
emptiness[2]	0
fatigability[1]	15
fatigability[2]	14
fears[1]	4
fears[2]	5
helplessness[1]	2
helplessness[2]	1
hopelessness[1]	0
hopelessness[2]	0
irritability[1]	7
irritability[2]	5
loss if interest[1]	1
loss if interest[2]	3
loss of activity[1]	4

Symptom	%
loss of activity[2]	5
loss of libido[1]	36
loss of libido[2]	46
loss of motivation[1]	2
loss of motivation[2]	3
loss of weight[1]	1
loss of weight[2]	1
low self esteem[1]	2
low self esteem[2]	6
negative feelings toward self[1]	0
negative feelings toward self[2]	0
nihilistic delusions[1]	0
nihilistic delusions[2]	0
other delusions[1]	0
other delusions[2]	0
other hallucinations[1]	0
other hallucinations[2]	0
pains[1]	19
pains[2]	22
pessimism[1]	1
pessimism[2]	3
poor memory[1]	5
poor memory[2]	6
psychomotor agitation[1]	6
psychomotor agitation[2]	5
restlessness[1]	4
restlessness[2]	4
restlessness[1]	1
restlessness[2]	2
retardation[1]	4
retardation[2]	4
rumination of problems[1]	7
rumination of problems[2]	5
sad expression[1]	1
sad expression[2]	3

scarcity of gestures[1]	1
scarcity of gestures[2]	3
self blame and criticism[1]	0
self blame and criticism[2]	0
sense of failure[1]	0
sense of failure[2]	1
sleep disturbances[1]	36
sleep disturbances[2]	43
sleep disturbances[1]	0
sleep disturbances[2]	0
slow movements[1]	7
slow movements[2]	4
slow speech[1]	5
slow speech[2]	4
somatic delusions[1]	0
somatic delusions[2]	0

stooping posture[1]	1
stooping posture[2]	1
suicidal ideas[1]	1
suicidal ideas[2]	4
suicidal impulses[1]	1
suicidal impulses[2]	0
uselessness[1]	2
uselessness[2]	2
visual hallucinations[1]	0
visual hallucinations[2]	0
weight loss[1]	0
weight loss[2]	1
worry[1]	2
worry[2]	3

Kivela & Pahkela (1988)
n = 330
Diagnostic Criteria:
Gender: [1]138/[2]192
Age: 60-69
Race:

Population Setting: community
Nationality: Finland
Other Sample Characteristics:
Method of Reporting: physician's
assessment
Timeframe: current

Symptom	%
crying[1]	1
crying[2]	0
psychomotor agitation[1]	7
psychomotor agitation[2]	6
sad expression[1]	1
sad expression[2]	5
scarcity of gestures[1]	0

Symptom	%
scarcity of gestures[2]	1
slow movement[1]	4
slow movements[2]	2
stooping posture[1]	1
stooping posture[2]	0
weight loss[1]	0

Kivela & Pahkela (1988)
n = 330
Diagnostic Criteria:
Gender: [1]138/[2]192
Age: 70+
Race:

Population Setting: community
Nationality: Finland
Other Sample Characteristics:
Method of Reporting: physician's
assessment
Timeframe: current

Symptom	%
crying[1]	0
crying[2]	2
psychomotor agitation[1]	4

Symptom	%
psychomotor agitation[2]	4
sad expression[1]	0
sad expression[2]	1

scarcity of gestures[1]	3
scarcity of gestures[2]	4
slow movements[1]	9
slow movements[2]	5

slow speech[1]	9
stooping posture[1]	0
stooping posture[2]	1
weight loss[1]	0

Nyhlin, Ford, Eastwood, et al. (1993)
n = 113
Diagnostic Criteria:
Gender: 46/67
Age: 45 (15)
Race:

Population Setting: general practice patients
Nationality: UK
Other Sample Characteristics:
Method of Reporting: self-report
Timeframe: 6 months

Symptom	%
dizziness	2
dysmenorrhoea	33
dyspareunia	6
heart pounding	8
paraesthesiae	10

Symptom	%
poor sleep	27
tiredness	48
tummy butterflies	6
urinary frequency	25

O'Keefe, Talley, Zinsmeister, et al. (1995)
n = 530
Diagnostic Criteria:
Gender: [1]270/[2]260
Age: 65+
Race: [1]270/0/0/0/0; [2]260/0/0/0/0

Population Setting: community
Nationality: US
Other Sample Characteristics:
Method of Reporting: self-report
Timeframe: 1 year

Symptoms	%
chronic constipation[1]	22.7
chronic constipation[2]	32.6
chronic diarrhea[1]	18.7
chronic diarrhea[2]	19.7

Symptoms	%
fecal incontinence[1]	8.1
fecal incontinence[2]	7.9
frequent abdominal pain[1]	21.1
frequent abdominal pain[2]	31.0

Sloane, Blazer, & George (1989)
n = 1620
Diagnostic Criteria:
Gender:
Age: [1]60-64; [2]65-69; [3]70-74; [4]75-79; [5]80-84; [6]85+
Race:
Population Setting: community

Nationality:
Other Sample Characteristics:
severity criteria: resulting in a physician visit, in taking a medication more than once, or interfering with activities "a lot"
Method of Reporting: self-report
Timeframe: 1 year

Symptom	%
dizziness[1]	17.8
dizziness[2]	15.6
dizziness[3]	18.7

Symptom	%
dizziness[4]	20.1
dizziness[5]	23.8
dizziness[6]	21.3

Bowling (1990)
n = 662
Diagnostic Criteria:
Gender: 126/536
Age: 85+
Race:

Population Setting: community
Nationality: UK
Other Sample Characteristics:
Method of Reporting: self-report
Timeframe: current

Symptom	%
abdominal pain	29
aches/pains/stiff muscles/joints	84
alternate constipation/loose	11
chest pain/heart trouble	34
constipation	39
depressed/suicidal thoughts	15
feelings of anxiety	29

Symptom	%
forgetfulness	44
giddiness	50
headache	28
loss of appetite	30
nerves/stress depression	62
piles	18
poor perceived health and feelings of poor self worth	49
sleeplessness	61
urinary incontinence	40

Judd, Rapaport, Paulus, et al. (1994)
n = 9160
Diagnostic Criteria:
Gender: 4195/4965
Age: 18+
Race: 5111/2125/1392

Population Setting: community
Nationality: US
Other Sample Characteristics:
Method of Reporting: structured interview
Timeframe: 1 month

Symptoms	%
a lot more trouble concentrating	9.0
increased appetite; gained as much as two pounds per week	9.5
less interest in sex than usual	9.5

Symptom	%
sleeping too much	8.7
tired out all the time	22.8
trouble falling asleep, staying asleep, waking up early	33.7

Porter, Penny, Russell, et al. (1996)
n = 6096
Diagnostic Criteria:
Gender: 0/6096

Age: 45-54
Race:
Population Setting: community
Nationality: UK

Other Sample Characteristics:
Method of Reporting: postal
questionnaire

Timeframe: 6 months

Symptom	%
aching/painful joints	67
anxiety	58
concentration/memory problems	60
depression	51
depression	51
dizziness	37
dry/sore vagina	34
feeling unable to cope	43

Symptom	%
headaches	60
hot flushes	57
irritability	72
night sweats	55
nocturia	48
palpitations	37
sleep problems	66
sore breasts	51

Ninomiya, Ohmori, Hashimoto, et al.
(1995)
$\underline{n} = 142$
Diagnostic Criteria:
Gender:
Age: 20-89
Race:

Population Setting: community
Nationality: Japan
Other Sample Characteristics:
Method of Reporting: neurological
exam
Timeframe: current

Symptom	%
ataxia	6
dysarthia	2
hypoesthesia	20

Symptom	%
impairment of hearing	13
visual change	1

McKinlay & Jeffreys (1974)
$\underline{n} = 638$
Diagnostic Criteria:
Gender: 0/638
Age: 45-54
Race:

Population Setting: community
Nationality: UK
Other Sample Characteristics:
Method of Reporting: postal survey
Timeframe: 1 year

Symptom	%
depression	50.1
dizzy spells	3.05
headaches	40.8
hot flushes	49.8
night sweats	40.8

Symptom	%
no symptoms	8.6
palpitations	35.0
sleeplessness	36.0
weight increase	47.5

Pham, Grisco, Freeman (1997)
n = 68
Diagnostic Criteria:
Gender: 0/68
Age: [1]45.6-46.7; [2]46.5-47.5
Race: [1]0/33/0/0/0/0; [2]35/0/0/0/0/0

Population Setting: community
Nationality:
Other Sample Characteristics:
Method of Reporting:
Timeframe: 2 months

Symptom	%
menstrual irregularity[1]	50.0
menstrual irregularity[2]	33.3

Kuh, Wadsworth, & Hardy (1997)
n = 1498
Diagnostic Criteria:
Gender: 0/1498
Age: 47
Race:

Population Setting: community
Nationality: UK
Other Sample Characteristics:
Method of Reporting: postal survey
Timeframe: 12 months

Symptom	%
aches and pains	59.7
anxiety and depression	52.0
breast tenderness	43.5
cold/night sweats	26.2
difficulties with intercourse	13.0
dizziness	27.8
feelings of panic	24.4
forgetfulness	44.3
hair loss	8.0
hot flushes	31.4

Symptom	%
irritability	54.8
palpitations	28.7
pins and needles	25.6
severe headaches	31.8
skin crawling sensations	14.4
skin wrinkling	18.5
tearfulness	41.8
trouble sleeping	49.4
urinary frequency	26.5
vaginal dryness	19.9

Cottler, Compton, Mager, et al. (1992)
n = 215
Diagnostic Criteria:
Gender:
Age:
Race:

Population Setting: community
Nationality: US
Other Sample Characteristics: experienced traumatic event
Method of Reporting: structured interview
Timeframe: following trauma

Symptom	%
ashamed	5
avoidance	24
guardedness	26

Symptom	%
jumpiness	44
loss of interest	16
nightmares	41

sleep problems	38
social impairment	13

trouble concentrating	26

Hollander, Greenwald, Neville, et al.
(1996/97)
n = 13899
Diagnostic Criteria: DSM III
Gender: 5361/8538
Age: 18+
Race: 9294/3113/1016

Population Setting: community
Nationality: US
Other Sample Characteristics:
Method of Reporting: structured
interview
Timeframe: [1]lifetime; [2]current

Symptom	%
cognitive impairment[1]	3.9
mild cognitive impairment[1]	3.4

Symptom	%
suicide attempts[1]	0.9

Kinjo, Higashi, Nakano, et al. (1993)
n = 1144
Diagnostic Criteria:
Gender: 586/558
Age: [1]40+; [2]40-49; [3]50-59; [4]60-69;
[5]70-79; [6]80+
Race:

Population Setting: community
Nationality: Japan
Other Sample Characteristics:
Method of Reporting: self-report
Timeframe: current

Symptom	%
constriction of visual field[1]	5.2
constriction of visual field[2]	0.9
constriction of visual field[3]	3.8
constriction of visual field[4]	4.2
constriction of visual field[5]	7.1
constriction of visual field[6]	8.8
cramp[1]	13.5
cramp[2]	8.1
cramp[3]	8.6
cramp[4]	10.5
cramp[5]	20.8
cramp[6]	16.3
difficulty buttoning[1]	11.7

Symptom	%
difficulty buttoning[2]	1.8
difficulty buttoning[3]	4.5
difficulty buttoning[4]	6.3
difficulty buttoning[5]	15.5
difficulty buttoning[6]	32.5
difficulty hearing[1]	15.9
difficulty hearing[2]	5.4
difficulty hearing[3]	6.0
difficulty hearing[4]	8.8
difficulty hearing[5]	23.6
difficulty hearing[6]	36.9
difficulty speaking[1]	5.9
difficulty speaking[2]	3.6
difficulty speaking[3]	3.8
difficulty speaking[4]	2.8
difficulty speaking[5]	7.5
difficulty speaking[6]	13.1
dizziness[1]	7.5
dizziness[2]	3.6

dizziness[3]	7.1		low back pain[1]	66.2
dizziness[4]	6.7		low back pain[2]	59.5
dizziness[5]	8.1		low back pain[3]	65.8
dizziness[6]	11.3		low back pain[4]	66.7
dysesthesia of limbs[1]	28.9		low back pain[5]	70.2
dysesthesia of limbs[2]	18.9		low back pain[6]	64.4
dysesthesia of limbs[3]	27.1		ptyalism[1]	3.8
dysesthesia of limbs[4]	29.5		ptyalism[2]	0.9
dysesthesia of limbs[5]	29.8		ptyalism[3]	0.8
dysesthesia of limbs[6]	36.3		ptyalism[4]	2.8
fatigability[1]	36.3		ptyalism[5]	5.9
fatigability[2]	25.2		ptyalism[6]	8.8
fatigability[3]	27.8		stumbling[1]	20.5
fatigability[4]	28.1		stumbling[2]	0.9
fatigability[5]	41.9		stumbling[3]	9.4
fatigability[6]	50.0		stumbling[4]	13.7
forgetfulness[1]	34.4		stumbling[5]	28.9
forgetfulness[2]	19.8		stumbling[6]	47.5
forgetfulness[3]	25.2		tinnitus[1]	18.8
forgetfulness[4]	31.9		tinnitus[2]	14.3
forgetfulness[5]	23.6		tinnitus[3]	9.0
forgetfulness[6]	49.4		tinnitus[4]	12.4
hypoesthesia of limbs[1]	28.9		tinnitus[5]	11.6
hypoesthesia of limbs[2]	3.6		tinnitus[6]	18.0
hypoesthesia of limbs[3]	13.5		tremor[1]	6.2
hypoesthesia of limbs[4]	10.5		tremor[2]	0.9
hypoesthesia of limbs[5]	15.5		tremor[3]	1.9
hypoesthesia of limbs[6]	23.8		tremor[4]	3.5
hypoesthesia of mouth[1]	13.6		tremor[5]	8.7
hypoesthesia of mouth[2]	0.0		tremor[6]	16.9
hypoesthesia of mouth[3]	1.9		weakness[1]	16.9
hypoesthesia of mouth[4]	2.1		weakness[2]	7.2
hypoesthesia of mouth[5]	3.1		weakness[3]	6.4
hypoesthesia of mouth[6]	3.1		weakness[4]	11.2
incontinence[1]	6.1		weakness[5]	23.0
incontinence[2]	0.0		weakness[6]	38.3
incontinence[3]	0.8			
incontinence[4]	2.1			
incontinence[5]	7.5			
incontinence[6]	23.8			

Mittenberg, DiGiulio, & Perrin
(1989)
n = 223
Diagnostic Criteria:
Gender: 586/558

Age: 30.2 (9.9)
Race:
Population Setting: community
Nationality: US
Other Sample Characteristics:

Method of Reporting: self-report   Timeframe: current

Symptom	%
anxiety	24.2
blurry or double vision	8.1
concentration difficulty	13.5
depression	19.7
dizziness	7.2
fatigue	12.6
forgets appointment dates	20.2
forgets content of daily conversations	16.6
forgets directions	24.2
forgets faces of new acquaintances	16
forgets groceries	28.3
forgets names of new acquaintances	10.1
forgets recent telephone conversations	8.5
forgets store locations in shopping centers	20

Symptom	%
forgets television news stories	12.1
forgets where car was parked	32
forgets where they went today	4.9
forgets who telephoned recently	5.8
forgets who they saw yesterday	12.1
forgets why they entered room	26.5
forgets yesterday's breakfast	26.9
forgets yesterday's newspaper articles	17
gets lost when driving	9
headache	12.5
irritability	15.7
loses car keys	31
loses items around the house	17
loses pocketbook or wallet	16.6
sensitivity to bright light	13.9
trouble thinking	6.3

Demallie, Cottler, & Compton (1995)
n = 170
Diagnostic Criteria: DSM-III
Gender: 82/88
Age: 38.02
Race: 103/0/0/0/0/67
Population Setting: community

Nationality: US
Other Sample Characteristics: used illicit drugs more than 5 times
Method of Reporting: structured interview
Timeframe: lifetime

Symptom	%
arrests	14.9
blackouts	34.1
couldn't do work well without drinking	4.8
establishes rules to control drinking	10.1
family objected	20.6
fights	23.2

Symptom	%
friends or doctor said drinking too much	15.5
job or school troubles	8.3
trouble driving	11.9
wanted to stop drinking but couldn't	11.8
withdrawal shakes	5.92

Bowler, Huel, Mergler, et al. (1996)
n = 230
Diagnostic Criteria:

Gender: [1]5/57; [2]35/55; [3]30/48
Age: [1]43.9(10.86); [2]44.4(13.00); [3]43.7(14.49)

Race: [1]0/0/62/0/0/0; [2]90/0/0/0/0/0;
[3]0/78/0/0/0/0
Population Setting: community
Nationality:

Other Sample Characteristics:
Method of Reporting: self-report
Timeframe: 1 month

Symptom	%
blurred vision[1]	21.0
blurred vision[2]	16.9
blurred vision[3]	32.1
change in personality[1]	12.9
change in personality[2]	11.2
change in personality[3]	37.2
confusion/lost[1]	4.8
confusion/lost[2]	12.6
confusion/lost[3]	44.9
dark vision[1]	4.8
dark vision[2]	0.0
dark vision[3]	11.5
diarrhea[1]	9.7
diarrhea[2]	14.9
diarrhea[3]	13.0
difficulty concentrating[1]	29.0
difficulty concentrating[2]	23.6
difficulty concentrating[3]	46.2
difficulty driving[1]	3.2
difficulty driving[2]	4.0
difficulty driving[3]	11.7
difficulty sleeping[1]	25.8
difficulty sleeping[2]	34.8
difficulty sleeping[3]	41.0
fainting[1]	4.8
fainting[2]	2.3
fainting[3]	2.3
feel anxious[1]	22.6
feel anxious[2]	38.2
feel anxious[3]	50.6
feel depressed[1]	29.0
feel depressed[2]	36.4
feel depressed[3]	60.3
feel irritable[1]	24.2
feel irritable[2]	46.1
feel irritable[3]	51.5
headaches minimum 1 day per week[1]	22.6
headaches minimum 1 day per week[2]	30.3

Symptom	%
headaches minimum 1 day per week[3]	34.6
heart palpitations[1]	8.1
heart palpitations[2]	17.0
heart palpitations[3]	19.5
incoordination[1]	6.5
incoordination[2]	13.5
incoordination[3]	21.8
joint pain or swelling[1]	8.1
joint pain or swelling[2]	17.0
joint pain or swelling[3]	26.0
lightheaded[1]	9.7
lightheaded[2]	19.1
lightheaded[3]	42.3
loss of smell[1]	8.1
loss of smell[2]	6.7
loss of smell[3]	10.3
loss of strength in arms/hand[1]	19.7
loss of strength in arms/hand[2]	15.7
loss of strength in arms/hand[3]	23.4
loss strength in legs/feet[1]	19.4
loss strength in legs/feet[2]	11.4
loss strength in legs/feet[3]	25.6
lower alcohol tolerance[1]	6.7
lower alcohol tolerance[2]	11.2
lower alcohol tolerance[3]	15.4
muscle twitching[1]	11.3
muscle twitching[2]	30.3
muscle twitching[3]	37.2
nausea, not food[1]	1.6
nausea, not food[2]	9.1
nausea, not food[3]	17.9
numbness/tingling fingers minimum 1 per day[1]	12.9
numbness/tingling fingers minimum 1 per day[2]	11.6
numbness/tingling fingers	24.4

minimum 1 per day[3]	
perspiring, no reason[1]	8.1
perspiring, no reason[2]	7.9
perspiring, no reason[3]	21.8
skin rashes[1]	18.0
skin rashes[2]	3.4
skin rashes[3]	11.0
sleeping more[1]	11.3
sleeping more[2]	20.0
sleeping more[3]	33.3
stomach cramps or pain[1]	9.7
stomach cramps or pain[2]	16.6
stomach cramps or pain[3]	25.6
tightness in chest[1]	9.7
tightness in chest[2]	10.3
tightness in chest[3]	17.9

tired more easily[1]	35.5
tired more easily[2]	46.7
tired more easily[3]	67.0
tremors[1]	19.7
tremors[2]	5.7
tremors[3]	20.8
trouble remembering[1]	37.1
trouble remembering[2]	37.1
trouble remembering[3]	47.4
weight loss, excluding dieting[1]	8.2
weight loss, excluding dieting[2]	4.5
weight loss, excluding dieting[3]	16.7

Blakely, Howard, Sosich, et al.
(1991)
n = 104
Diagnostic Criteria:
Gender: 32/72
Age: 39.7 (16-60)

Race:
Population Setting: outpatient clinic
Nationality: New Zealand
Other Sample Characteristics:
Method of Reporting: BDI
Timeframe:

Symptom	%
mild depression	12.5
moderate depression	15.2
severe depression	0.0

Wessely, Chalder, Hirsch, et al.
(1996)
n = 193
Diagnostic Criteria:
Gender:
Age: 18-34

Race:
Population Setting: community
Nationality: UK
Other Sample Characteristics:
Method of Reporting: self-report
Timeframe: since onset

Symptom	%
back pain	36
chest pain	8
constipation	14
daytime drowsiness	41
diarrhea	14
difficulty in urinating	3
dizziness	12

Symptom	%
double vision	4
dry mouth	20
eyestrain	23
faster breathing than normal	5
fever/chills	14
headaches	47

inability to breathe deeply enough	9
increased sensitivity to light	11
increased sensitivity to noise	13
joint pain	19
light-headedness	13
muscle weakness	14
myalgia	23
nausea	21
neuropsychological disturbance	23
pain in eyes	13

pain on urinating	3
palpitations	15
post exertion malaise	22
ringing in ears	7
shortness of breath at rest	4
sleep disturbance	31
sore glands	7
sore throat	21
stiffness	22
stomach pain	25
tingling in fingers or arms	13
tingling in legs or feet	8
tremor	6
urinating more often	12

Little, Snell, Rosenfeld, et al. (1990)
n = 80
Diagnostic Criteria:
Gender:
Age: infants
Race:

Population Setting: community
Nationality:
Other Sample Characteristics:
Method of Reporting: physical exam
Timeframe: at birth

Symptom	%
eyelid ptosis	0
facies	0
flattened nasal bridges	0

Symptom	%
low-set ears	0
short noses	0
short-neck	0

Raja, Feehan, Stanton, et al. (1992)
n = 384
Diagnostic Criteria:
Gender: 0/384
Age: 15
Race:

Population Setting: community
Nationality: New Zealand
Other Sample Characteristics:
Method of Reporting: self-report
Timeframe: [1]before menstruation;
[2]during menstruation

Symptom	%
argue more often[1]	10.7
argue more often[2]	10.4
avoiding people[1]	1.3
avoiding people[2]	2.6
backache[1]	7.0
backache[2]	7.6
constipation[1]	1.0
constipation[2]	1.3
crave special food[1]	4.7

Symptom	%
crave special food[2]	3.9
diarrhea[1]	0.3
diarrhea[2]	0.5
eat more than usual[1]	5.7
eat more than usual[2]	5.7
fainting or blackouts[1]	0.5
fainting or blackouts[2]	0.8
feel like crying[1]	3.4
feel like crying[2]	2.6

feel relaxed[1]	3.6
feel relaxed[2]	3.4
feel sad & blue[1]	5.5
feel sad & blue[2]	6.0
feel tired[1]	11.5
feel tired[2]	13.5
feeling irritable[1]	14.3
feeling irritable[2]	12.2
forgetful[1]	1.6
forgetful[2]	1.6
have small accidents[1]	0.8
have small accidents[2]	0.5
headache[1]	4.7
headache[2]	6.0
more happy and contented[1]	3.4
more happy and contented[2]	3.4
nausea & vomiting[1]	3.4
nausea & vomiting[2]	3.6
pain elsewhere in chest[1]	1.0

pain elsewhere in chest[2]	1.3
pains in limbs[1]	2.9
pains in limbs[2]	2.9
pallor[1]	3.6
pallor[2]	4.2
poor concentration[1]	3.1
poor concentration[2]	4.2
poor coordination[1]	1.0
poor coordination[2]	0.8
stomach cramps[1]	15.4
stomach cramps[2]	17.7
tender breasts[1]	3.1
tender breasts[2]	2.3
use time efficiently[1]	4.2
use time efficiently[2]	3.4
want to be alone[1]	3.1
want to be alone[2]	3.4

Yu, Hsu, Gladen, et al. (1991)
n = 118
Diagnostic Criteria:
Gender:
Age: few months-just under 7 years
Race:

Population Setting: community
Nationality: Taiwan
Other Sample Characteristics:
Method of Reporting: neurological exam
Timeframe: current

Symptom	%
developmental or psychomotor delay	2
speech problem	3

Koegel & Burnham (1988)
n = 10108
Diagnostic Criteria:
Gender:
Age: 16-64
Race:

Population Setting: community
Nationality: UK
Other Sample Characteristics:
Method of Reporting: structured interview
Timeframe: 1 week

Symptom	%
fatigue	27
irritability	22

Symptom	%
sleep problems	25
worry	20

Koegel & Burnham (1988)
n = 2283
Diagnostic Criteria:
Gender:
Age: 18-65
Race:

Population Setting: community
Nationality: Sweden
Other Sample Characteristics:
Method of Reporting: psychiatric
interview
Timeframe: 12 months

Symptom	%
"consolation eating", weight increase	4.2
compulsions	1.6
depression	17.6
dizziness in form of unsteadiness and insecurity	6.7
general feeling of tension	12.2
hallucinations	0.5
mental, psychosomatic symptoms, total	66.7
migraine	5.1
obsessions	1.8

Symptom	%
phobias	8.7
"psychosomatic back-joint symptoms"	24.0
"psychosomatic breathing difficulties"	3.2
"psychosomatic cardiac irregularities"	17.5
"psychosomatic gastrointestinal symptoms"	23.6
restlessness, anxiety attacks	15
sleep problems	17.1
stammering	0.9
tension headache	17.0

Yuk, Jugdutt, Cumming, et al. (1990)
n = 133
Diagnostic Criteria:
Gender: 0/133
Age: 33.6 (0.8); 19-52
Race:
Population Setting: community

Nationality: Canada
Other Sample Characteristics:
Method of Reporting: self report
questionnaire
Timeframe: During premenstrual
period

Symptom	%
autonomic physical	16.5
fatigue	25.6
general physical discomfort	61.7

Symptom	%
impaired social function	39.1
impulsive	27.8
increased wellbeing	12.8
water retention	53.4

Frost Steketee Krause, et al. (1995)
n = 45
Diagnostic Criteria:
Gender: 0/45
Age: 18-22
Race:

Population Setting: college
undergraduate
Nationality: US
Other Sample Characteristics:
Method of Reporting: self-report
checklist

Timeframe:

Symptom	%
being bother by sticky substances	22.2
compulsions checking	28.9
concerns about harming others	15.6
concerns with arranging, ordering, symmetry	17.7

Symptom	%
fear of forgetting	22.2
hoarding compulsion	20.0
list making	17.7
need to tell ask, confess	24.4

Bulpitt, Dollery, & Carne (1974)
n = 945
Diagnostic Criteria:
Gender: [1]0/249; [2]0/226; [3]0/430; [4]0/40
Age: [1]32-69; [3]55.7; [4]48.5
Race:

Population Setting: community
Nationality: UK
Other Sample Characteristics:
Method of Reporting: postal survey
Timeframe:

Symptom	%
blurring of vision[1]	22.7
blurring of vision[2]	18.4
blurring of vision[3]	20.2
blurring of vision[4]	22.9
change of therapy[1]	26.0
change of therapy[2]	14.4
depression[1]	35.8
depression[2]	22.4
depression[3]	28.3
depression[4]	28.3
diarrhea[1]	30.2
diarrhea[2]	30.6
diarrhea[3]	28.7
diarrhea[4]	28.7
dry mouth[1]	41.9
dry mouth[2]	38.4
dry mouth[3]	41.9
dry mouth[4]	41.9
failure of ejaculation[3]	26.4
failure of ejaculation[4]	26.4
headache[1]	21.1
headache[2]	9.5
headache[3]	13.8
headache[4]	31.7

Symptom	%
impotence[3]	42.8
impotence[4]	42.8
nocturia[1]	1.19
nocturia[2]	1.09
nocturia[3]	0.0
nocturia[4]	0.0
postural hypertension[1]	34.4
postural hypertension[2]	32.6
postural hypertension[3]	33.4
postural hypertension[4]	36.1
sleepiness[1]	52.5
sleepiness[2]	50.0
sleepiness[3]	50.1
sleepiness[4]	62.5
slow walking pace[1]	35.6
slow walking pace[2]	38.1
slow walking pace[3]	36.6
slow walking pace[4]	37.5
weak limbs[1]	26.9
weak limbs[2]	25.9
weak limbs[3]	24.3
weak limbs[4]	46.2

Frost, Krause, & Steketee (1996)
n = 45
Diagnostic Criteria:
Gender: 0/45
Age: 18-22
Race:

Population Setting: college
undergraduates
Nationality: US
Other Sample Characteristics:
Method of Reporting: self-report
checklist
Timeframe:

Symptom	%
hoarding compulsions	33
hoarding obsessions	30

Woods, Most, Dery, et al. (1982)
n = 179
Diagnostic Criteria:
Gender: 0/179
Age: 18-35
Race: 120/59/0/0/0/0
Population Setting: community

Nationality: US
Other Sample Characteristics:
Method of Reporting: structured
interview
Timeframe: [1]last menstrual period;
[2]last premenstrual period

Symptom	%
mild/moderate anxiety[1]	20.2
mild/moderate anxiety[2]	27.0
mild/moderate backache[1]	25.1
mild/moderate backache[2]	16.8
mild/moderate cramps[1]	36.3
mild/moderate cramps[2]	24.6
mild/moderate crying[1]	15.6
mild/moderate crying[2]	19.6
mild/moderate depression[1]	29.7
mild/moderate depression[2]	29.7
mild/moderate fatigue[1]	40.2
mild/moderate fatigue[2]	28.5
mild/moderate headaches[1]	27.4
mild/moderate headaches[2]	27.4
mild/moderate irritability[1]	37.8
mild/moderate irritability[2]	44.2
mild/moderate lower work and school performance[1]	14.5
mild/moderate lower work and school performance[2]	11.7
mild/moderate mood swings[1]	43.0
mild/moderate mood swings[2]	46.5

Symptom	%
mild/moderate painful breasts[1].	25.1
mild/moderate painful breasts[2].	27.9
mild/moderate skin disorder[1]	30.2
mild/moderate skin disorder[2]	32.4
mild/moderate swelling[1]	34.3
mild/moderate swelling[2]	39.5
mild/moderate taking of naps[1]	22.9
mild/moderate taking of naps[2]	17.3
mild/moderate tension[1]	37.8
mild/moderate tension[2]	34.3
mild/moderate weight gain[1]	30.9
mild/moderate weight gain[2]	40.2
severe/disabling anxiety[1]	3.9
severe/disabling anxiety[2]	3.4
severe/disabling	6.1

backache[1]	
severe/disabling backache[2]	5.0
severe/disabling cramps[1]	16.8
severe/disabling cramps[2]	6.1
severe/disabling crying[1]	2.8
severe/disabling crying[2]	4.5
severe/disabling depression[1]	5.2
severe/disabling depression[2]	7.0
severe/disabling fatigue[1]	7.3
severe/disabling fatigue[2]	3.9
severe/disabling headaches[1]	7.3
severe/disabling headaches[2]	7.3
severe/disabling irritability[1]	11.0
severe/disabling irritability[2]	12.2
severe/disabling lower work and school performance[1]	3.9
severe/disabling lower work and school	3.4

performance[2]	
severe/disabling mood swings[1]	3.5
severe/disabling mood swings[2]	4.7
severe/disabling painful breasts[1].	4.7
severe/disabling painful breasts[2].	7.6
severe/disabling skin disorder[1]	3.4
severe/disabling skin disorder[2]	6.7
severe/disabling swelling[1]	4.7
severe/disabling swelling[2]	5.2
severe/disabling taking of knaps[1]	3.4
severe/disabling taking of naps[2]	1.1
severe/disabling tension[1]	5.8
severe/disabling tension[2]	7.6
severe/disabling weight gain[1]	2.2
severe/disabling weight gain[2]	5.6

Ardila & Bateman (1995)
n = 1,816
Diagnostic Criteria:
Gender: 913/903
Age:
Race:

Population Setting: university students
Nationality: Colombia
Other Sample Characteristics:
Method of Reporting: questionnaire
Timeframe:

Symptom	%
confusional spells	1.5
environmental distortion	1.3
impending doom	2.9
mental decline	2.4
paranoia	2.0

Symptom	%
religiousness	6.0
somnambulism	11.8
suicidal ideation	1.9
suicide attempts	5.6

Toole, Lefkowitz, Chambless, et al. (1996)
n = 12,205
Diagnostic Criteria:
Gender: 5435/6770

Age: 45-64
Race:
Population Setting: longitudinal atherosclerosis study participants
Nationality: US

Other Sample Characteristics: sudden
onset of symptoms

Method of Reporting: self report
questionnaire
Timeframe: lifetime

Symptom	%
dizziness Imbalance	35.9
double vision	4.5
numbness	16.0

Symptom	%
speech dysfunction	2.6
visual impairment	6.0
weakness paralysis	2.3

Vetter, Jones, & Victor (1981)
n = 1,280
Diagnostic Criteria:
Gender:
Age: [1]70-74; [2]75-79; [3]80-84; [31]85+
Race:

Population Setting: community
Nationality: UK
Other Sample Characteristics:
Method of Reporting: questionnaire
Timeframe: current

Symptom	%
daily incontinence[1]	5.9
daily incontinence[2]	12.3
daily incontinence[3]	21.0
daily Incontinence[31]	85.8
less than daily incontinence[1]	12.9

Symptom	%
less than daily incontinence[2]	21.3
less than daily incontinence[3]	53.2
less than daily incontinence[31]	75.2

Hill, Standen, & Tattersfield (1989)
n = 3805
Diagnostic Criteria:
Gender:
Age: 5-11
Race:

Population Setting: public school
students
Nationality: UK
Other Sample Characteristics:
Method of Reporting: parental
questionnaire
Timeframe: [1]lifetime; [2]1 year

Symptom	%
bronchitis[1]	5.1
night cough[2]	11.5

Symptom	%
wheezing cough[2]	9.6
wheezing[1]	17.5

Warner & Bancroft (1990)
n = 5457
Diagnostic Criteria:
Gender: 0/5457
Age:
Race:

Population Setting: women's
magazine readers
Nationality: UK
Other Sample Characteristics:
Method of Reporting: women's
magazine survey

Timeframe: [1]during one week of prior to last menstrual period; [2]during last menstrual period; [3]during last week menstrual period

Symptom	%
acne[1]	10
acne[2]	1
acne[3]	2
backache[1]	9
backache[2]	8
backache[3]	1
change in bowel habits[1]	9
change in bowel habits[2]	6
change in bowel habits[3]	1
clumsiness[1]	20
clumsiness[2]	2
clumsiness[3]	1
craving for sweet foods[1]	25
craving for sweet foods[2]	2
craving for sweet foods[3]	2
difficulty in sleeping[1]	11
difficulty in sleeping[2]	2
difficulty in sleeping[3]	2
easily upset[1]	41
easily upset[2]	3
easily upset[3]	3
feel bad about myself[1]	28
feel bad about myself[2]	3
feel bad about myself[3]	4
feel bloated in the abdomen[1]	33
feel bloated in the abdomen[2]	5
feel bloated in the abdomen[3]	1
feel depressed[1]	39
feel depressed[2]	3
feel depressed[3]	3
feeling tense[1]	35
feeling tense[2]	3
feeling tense[3]	3
general aches and pains[1]	10
general aches and pains[2]	4

Symptom	%
general aches and pains[3]	1
get angry for no good reason[1]	47
get angry for no good reason[2]	2
get angry for no good reason[3]	3
headaches[1]	15
headaches[2]	5
headaches[3]	3
hot flashes cold sweats[1]	8
hot flashes cold sweats[2]	3
hot flashes cold sweats[3]	1
irritable[1]	43
irritable[2]	3
irritable[3]	3
mood swings[1]	34
mood swings[2]	2
mood swings[3]	4
nausea sickness[1]	6
nausea sickness[2]	4
nausea sickness[3]	1
passing water frequently[1]	13
passing water frequently[2]	7
passing water frequently[3]	3
period type pains[1]	9
period type pains[2]	23
period type pains[3]	1
poor concentration[1]	22
poor concentration[2]	3
poor concentration[3]	2
tender breasts[1]	29
tender breasts[2]	1
tender breasts[3]	1
violent feelings[1]	24
violent feelings[2]	1
violent feelings[3]	2

Rubin, Morris, & Berg (1987)
<u>n</u> = 58
Diagnostic Criteria:

Gender: 28/30
Age: 71.7 (4.9); 64-83
Race:

Population Setting: women's
magazine readers
Nationality: UK
Other Sample Characteristics:

Method of Reporting: self & care
giver report
Timeframe: current

Symptom	%
agitated	5
passive	0
passive/agitated	0
passive/agitated/self centered	0

Symptom	%
passive/self centered	0
self centered	3

Hale, Perkins, May, et al. (1986)
n = 3067
Diagnostic Criteria:
Gender: 1140/1927
Age: [1]65-69; [2]70-74; [3]75-79; [4]80-84; [5]84+
Race:

Population Setting: community
members participating in a health
screening program
Nationality: US
Other Sample Characteristics: all
women
Method of Reporting: questionnaire
Timeframe: current

Symptom	%
blacking out[1]	3.0
blacking out[2]	3.7
blacking out[3]	6.5
blacking out[4]	5.8
blacking out[5]	13.6
blood in stool[1]	4.3
blood in stool[2]	2.4
blood in stool[3]	1.6
blood in stool[4]	3.5
blood in stool[5]	3.5
brief speech loss[1]	1.8
brief speech loss[2]	1.3
brief speech loss[3]	2.1
brief speech loss[4]	2.3
brief speech loss[5]	3.3
brief vision loss[1]	5.2
brief vision loss[2]	5.7
brief vision loss[3]	5.2
brief vision loss[4]	7.2
brief vision loss[5]	11.2
burning on urination[1]	6.1
burning on urination[2]	4.9
burning on urination[3]	5.5

Symptom	%
burning on urination[4]	8.1
burning on urination[5]	10.3
change of voice[1]	1.8
change of voice[2]	2.7
change of voice[3]	5.0
change of voice[4]	10.4
change of voice[5]	7.0
chest discomfort with exercise[1]	14.2
chest discomfort with exercise[2]	11.8
chest discomfort with exercise[3]	16.1
chest discomfort with exercise[4]	16.5
chest discomfort with exercise[5]	12.9
chest discomfort with tension/anxiety[1]	21.7
chest discomfort with tension/anxiety[2]	15.9
chest discomfort with tension/anxiety[3]	16.4

chest discomfort with tension/anxiety[4]	16.0	walking[5]	
chest discomfort with tension/anxiety[5]	12.1	pain in hands/feet/legs with exposure to cold[1]	12.0
coughed up blood in last year[1]	0.3	pain in hands/feet/legs with exposure to cold[2]	10.4
coughed up blood in last year[2]	0.6	pain in hands/feet/legs with exposure to cold[3]	12.7
coughed up blood in last year[3]	0.4	pain in hands/feet/legs with exposure to cold[4]	13.8
coughed up blood in last year[4]	0.8	pain in hands/feet/legs with exposure to cold[5]	19.1
coughed up blood in last year[5]	0.0	parosxymal[1]	4.6
dizziness[1]	8.8	parosxymal[2]	5.3
dizziness[2]	11.8	parosxymal[3]	5.0
dizziness[3]	13.8	parosxymal[4]	3.8
dizziness[4]	16.0	parosxymal[5]	5.9
dizziness[5]	18.3	problems swallowing[1]	3.3
feet/ legs become cold with exposure to cold[1]	26.6	problems swallowing[2]	4.9
feet/ legs become cold with exposure to cold[2]	23.8	problems swallowing[3]	5.0
feet/ legs become cold with exposure to cold[3]	29.6	problems swallowing[4]	9.2
feet/ legs become cold with exposure to cold[4]	34.0	problems swallowing[5]	13.5
feet/ legs become cold with exposure to cold[5]	46.3	recurrent constipation[1]	23.7
frequent headaches[1]	14.9	recurrent constipation[2]	20.8
frequent headaches[2]	14.8	recurrent constipation[3]	30.2
frequent Headaches[3]	14.0	recurrent constipation[4]	32.4
frequent headaches[4]	13.0	recurrent constipation[5]	34.5
frequent headaches[5]	8.3	recurrent cough[1]	11.3
irregular heart beat[1]	24.2	recurrent cough[2]	13.4
irregular heart beat[2]	21.4	recurrent cough[3]	12.1
irregular heart beat[3]	23.3	recurrent cough[4]	22.7
irregular heart beat[4]	23.1	recurrent cough[5]	16.8
irregular heart beat[5]	31.0	recurrent pain in abdomen[1]	14.6
pain in calves/legs on walking[1]	11.0	recurrent pain in abdomen[2]	11.7
pain in calves/legs on walking[2]	11.7	recurrent pain in abdomen[3]	12.8
pain in calves/legs on walking[3]	11.9	recurrent pain in abdomen[4]	14.6
pain in calves/legs on walking[4]	17.7	recurrent pain in abdomen[5]	10.2
pain in calves/legs on	12.7	ringing ears[1]	22.2
		ringing ears[2]	22.4
		ringing ears[3]	21.3
		ringing ears[4]	24.8
		ringing ears[5]	20.8
		sensation of fainting or floating[1]	7.1

sensation of fainting or floating[2]	5.5
sensation of fainting or floating[3]	6.5
sensation of fainting or floating[4]	10.0
sensation of fainting or floating[5]	12.6
shortness of breath with less than normal exercise[1]	18.7
shortness in breath with less than normal exercise[2]	16.3
shortness in breath with less than normal exercise[3]	17.4
shortness in breath with less than normal exercise[4]	19.8
shortness in breath with less than normal exercise[5]	26.1

swollen feet or ankles[1]	29.2
swollen feet or ankles[2]	26.0
swollen feet or ankles[3]	31.3
swollen feet or ankles[4]	36.5
swollen feet or ankles[5]	43.1
transient numbness in arms/legs[1]	13.7
transient numbness in arms/legs[2]	11.1
transient numbness in arms/legs[3]	14.0
transient numbness in arms/legs[4]	13.4
transient numbness in arms/legs[5]	16.5

Hale, Perkins, May, et al. (1986)
n = 3067
Diagnostic Criteria:
Gender: 1140/1927
Age: [1]65-69; [2]70-74; [3]75-79; [4]80-84; [5]84+
Race:

Population Setting: community members participating in a health screening program
Nationality: US
Other Sample Characteristics: all men
Method of Reporting: questionnaire
Timeframe: current

Symptom	%
blacking out[1]	0.8
blacking out[2]	2.2
blacking out[3]	4.1
blacking out[4]	7.3
blacking out[5]	13.4
blood in stool[1]	1.6
blood in stool[2]	3.0
blood in stool[3]	3.0
blood in stool[4]	2.6
blood in stool[5]	3.0
brief speech loss[1]	2.4
brief speech loss[2]	1.0
brief speech loss[3]	1.2
brief speech loss[4]	2.6
brief speech loss[5]	9.1
brief vision loss[1]	4.8
brief vision loss[2]	3.5
brief vision loss[3]	4.4

Symptom	%
brief vision loss[4]	5.3
brief vision loss[5]	11.3
burning on urination[1]	5.7
burning on urination[2]	3.5
burning on urination[3]	3.2
burning on urination[4]	2.6
burning on urination[5]	6.1
change of voice[1]	0.8
change of voice[2]	2.7
change of voice[3]	6.2
change of voice[4]	4.6
change of voice[5]	6.2
chest discomfort with exercise[1]	11.8
chest discomfort with exercise[2]	13.8
chest discomfort with exercise[3]	16.1

chest discomfort with exercise[4]	20.0
chest discomfort with exercise[5]	10.7
chest discomfort with tension/anxiety[1]	10.5
chest discomfort with tension/anxiety[2]	12.3
chest discomfort with tension/anxiety[3]	13.5
chest discomfort with tension/anxiety[4]	19.4
chest discomfort with tension/anxiety[5]	16.2
coughed up blood in last year[1]	0.0
coughed up blood in last year[2]	1.7
coughed up blood in last year[3]	0.3
coughed up blood in last year[4]	0.0
coughed up blood in last year[5]	0.0
dizziness[1]	4.1
dizziness[2]	5.2
dizziness[3]	10.3
dizziness[4]	13.5
dizziness[5]	19.7
feet/ legs become cold with exposure to cold[1]	20.7
feet/ legs become cold with exposure to cold[2]	20.6
feet/ legs become cold with exposure to cold[3]	23.3
feet/ legs become cold with exposure to cold[4]	27.8
feet/ legs become cold with exposure to cold[5]	35.9
frequent headaches[1]	10.5
frequent headaches[2]	5.4
frequent headaches[3]	7.5
frequent headaches[4]	5.7
frequent headaches[5]	3.0
irregular heart beat[1]	18.2
irregular heart beat[2]	21.8
irregular heart beat[3]	26.8
irregular heart beat[4]	28.4

irregular heart beat[5]	33.9
pain in calves/legs on walking[1]	7.3
pain in calves/legs on walking[2]	11.9
pain in calves/legs on walking[3]	17.3
pain in calves/legs on walking[4]	21.2
pain in calves/legs on walking[5]	20.3
pain in hands/feet/legs with exposure to cold[1]	6.7
pain in hands/feet/legs with exposure to cold[2]	9.0
pain in hands/feet/legs with exposure to cold[3]	7.3
pain in hands/feet/legs with exposure to cold[4]	9.2
pain in hands/feet/legs with exposure to cold[5]	19.1
parosxymal[1]	2.4
parosxymal[2]	5.4
parosxymal[3]	4.1
parosxymal[4]	4.7
parosxymal[5]	4.6
problems swallowing[1]	2.4
problems swallowing[2]	3.2
problems swallowing[3]	3.8
problems swallowing[4]	6.7
problems swallowing[5]	10.6
recurrent constipation[1]	8.9
recurrent constipation[2]	8.8
recurrent constipation[3]	13.2
recurrent constipation[4]	26.1
recurrent constipation[5]	22.7
recurrent cough[1]	8.1
recurrent cough[2]	12.4
recurrent cough[3]	11.0
recurrent cough[4]	18.1
recurrent cough[5]	19.4
recurrent pain in abdomen[1]	4.9
recurrent pain in abdomen[2]	4.2
recurrent pain in abdomen[3]	7.3
recurrent pain in	5.7

abdomen[4]	
recurrent pain in abdomen[5]	10.6
ringing ears[1]	26.0
ringing ears[2]	23.3
ringing ears[3]	21.9
ringing ears[4]	20.6
ringing ears[5]	30.3
sensation of fainting or floating[1]	2.4
sensation of fainting or floating[2]	2.5
sensation of fainting or floating[3]	5.0
sensation of fainting or floating[4]	10.4
sensation of fainting or floating[5]	12.2
shortness of breath with less than normal exercise[1]	10.8
shortness in breath with less than normal exercise[2]	13.2

shortness in breath with less than normal exercise[3]	17.1
shortness in breath with less than normal exercise[4]	20.9
shortness in breath with less than normal exercise[5]	24.6
swollen feet or ankles[1]	1.7
swollen feet or ankles[2]	8.1
swollen feet or ankles[3]	10.7
swollen feet or ankles[4]	12.0
swollen feet or ankles[5]	26.6
transient numbness in arms/legs[1]	6.7
transient numbness in arms/legs[2]	9.7
transient numbness in arms/legs[3]	9.5
transient numbness in arms/legs[4]	12.8
transient numbness in arms/legs[5]	13.8

Breslau, Davis, & Andreski (1991)
n = 1,007
Diagnostic Criteria:
Gender: [1]386/[2]621
Age: 21-30
Race:

Population Setting: HMO members
Nationality: US
Other Sample Characteristics:
Method of Reporting: structured interview
Timeframe: 1 year

Symptom	%
migraine with aura[1]	1.3
migraine with aura[2]	6.0

Symptom	%
migraine without aura[1]	2.1
migraine without aura[2]	6.9

Breslau, Davis, & Andreski (1991)
n = 1,007
Diagnostic Criteria:
Gender: [1]386/[2]621
Age: 21-30
Race:

Population Setting: HMO members
Nationality: US
Other Sample Characteristics:
Method of Reporting: structured interview
Timeframe: lifetime

Symptom	%
migraine with aura[1]	3.4
migraine with aura[2]	7.4

Symptom	%
migraine without aura[1]	3.6
migraine without aura[2]	8.9

Breslau, Davis, & Andreski (1991)
n = 1,007
Diagnostic Criteria:
Gender:
Age: 21-30
Race: [1]813/0/0/0/0/0; [2]0/194/0/0/0/0

Population Setting: HMO members
Nationality: US
Other Sample Characteristics:
Method of Reporting: structured
interview
Timeframe: lifetime

Symptom	%
migraine with aura[1]	6.0
migraine with aura[2]	5.2

Symptom	%
migraine without aura[1]	6.9
migraine without aura[2]	6.7

Jolleys (1988)
n = 833
Diagnostic Criteria:
Gender: 0/833
Age:
Race:

Population Setting: general medicine
practice outpatients
Nationality: UK
Other Sample Characteristics:
Method of Reporting: postal survey
Timeframe:

Symptom	%
incontinence on climbing stairs	6
incontinence on coughing	24
incontinence on exercise	12
incontinence on laughing	16

Symptom	%
incontinence on lifting	8
incontinence on sneezing	11
incontinence with full bladder	20

Friedman, Asnis, Boeck, et al. (1987)
n = 380
Diagnostic Criteria:
Gender: 200/180
Age: 16.04 (1.2)
Race: 190/50/37/81/0/22

Population Setting: public school
students
Nationality: US
Other Sample Characteristics:
Method of Reporting: self-report
questionnaire
Timeframe:

Symptom	%
suicidal attempts	8.7
suicidal ideation	52.9

Price, North, Wessely, et al. (1992)
n = 13,538
Diagnostic Criteria:
Gender: 5,556/7,982

Age:
Race: 8118/3881/1366/0/0/0
Population Setting: community
Nationality: US

Other Sample Characteristics: Timeframe: lifetime
Method of Reporting: structured
interview

Symptom	%
50% reduction in activity	13.3
fatigue	23.7
general muscle weakness	8.7
generalized headache	20.5
muscle dyscontrol	18.0
neuropsychological complaints	81.2

Symptom	%
pain in joints	29.2
prolonged fatigue (>24 hours)	23.6
sleep disturbances	25.6
weight loss	14.4

Pfeffer, Lipkins, Plutchik, et al.   Nationality: US
(1984)   Other Sample Characteristics:
n = 75   Method of Reporting: [1]semi-
Diagnostic Criteria: structured interview of child; [2]semi-
Gender: 52/23   structured interview of mother; [3]semi-
Age: 12.1(.25)   structured interview of father
Race: 54/0/0/0/0/21   Timeframe: 6 months
Population Setting: school children

Symptom	%
suicidal ideation[1]	17.9
suicidal ideation[2]	10.7
suicidal ideation[3]	4.0
suicidal threats[1]	1.5
suicidal threats[2]	2.7

Symptom	%
suicidal threats[3]	0.0
suicide attempts[1]	0.0
suicide attempts[2]	1.3
suicide attempts[3]	1.3

Matthew, Weinman, & Mirabi (1981)   Population Setting: community
n = 51   Nationality: US
Diagnostic Criteria: Other Sample Characteristics:
Gender: Method of Reporting: self-report
Age: 29.6 (8.5); 18-65   questionnaire
Race: Timeframe:

Symptom	%
agitation	37.3
amenorrhea	2.9
blurred vision	7.9
chest pain	5.9
constipation	17.6
daytime drowsiness	51.0
delayed ejaculation	6.2

Symptom	%
difficulty in urination	4.0
dizziness	11.8
dry mouth	19.6
dry skin	39.2
excessive libido	0.0
excessive perspiration	13.7
excessive salivation	2.0

flushing	9.8
headaches	39.2
impaired concentration	29.4
impotency	0.0
lack of orgasm	11.4
loss of libido	6.0
polymenorrhea	2.9

premature ejaculation	0.0
rapid breathing	3.9
slurred speech	4.0
tinnitus	11.8
weakness	11.8
weight gain	23.5

Tashkin, Khalsa, Gorelick, et al.
(1992)
n = 43
Diagnostic Criteria:
Gender:
Age: 21-50

Race:
Population Setting: VA patients
Nationality: US
Other Sample Characteristics:
Method of Reporting:
Timeframe:

Symptom	%
acute brohchitic episodes	2.3
cough	0.0
shortness of breath	0.0

Symptom	%
sputum	2.3
wheezing	0.0

Sillanpaa (1983)
n = 3,784
Diagnostic Criteria:
Gender: [1]1,911/0; [2]0/1,873;
[3]1,911/1,873
Age: 21-50
Race:

Population Setting: school children
Nationality: Finland
Other Sample Characteristics:
Method of Reporting: self-report
questionnaire
Timeframe: 1 year

Symptom	%
classic migraine[1]	1.9
classic migraine[2]	6.5
common migraine[1]	6.2
common migraine[2]	8.0
headache[1]	80.0

Symptom	%
headache[2]	84.0
nausea/vomiting[3]	14.1
unilateral pain[3]	21.5
visual aura[3]	10.1

Talley, Zinsmeister, Schleck, et al.
(1992)
n = 835
Diagnostic Criteria:
Gender:
Age:

Race: 835/0/0/0/0/0
Population Setting: community
Nationality: US
Other Sample Characteristics:
Method of Reporting: postal survey
Timeframe: 1 year

Symptom	%
acid regurgitation once a month at least	11.3
acid regurgitation once a week at least	6.5
acid regurgitation several times a week or daily	3.6
anorexia	4.0
heartburn once a month at least	24.4
heartburn once a week at least	13.2
heartburn several times a week or daily	6.8

Symptom	%
nausea once a month at least	7.4
nausea once a week at least	3.4
nausea several times a week or daily	1.8
upper abdominal pain more than six times	15.7
upper abdominal pain once a week or more	8.2
upper abdominal pains	25.8
vomiting once a month at least	2.3

Talley, O'Keefe, Zinsmeister, et al. (1992)
n = 328
Diagnostic Criteria:
Gender:
Age: 65+

Race: 328/0/0/0/0/0
Population Setting: community
Nationality: US
Other Sample Characteristics:
Method of Reporting: postal survey
Timeframe: 1 year

Symptom	%
abdominal distension often	19.7
abdominal pain	41.2
abdominal pain more than six times	24.3
difficulty swallowing	11.2
enemas used	6.4
fecal incontinence more than once a week	3.7
feeling of an anal blockage often	15.2
feeling of incomplete evacuation often	25.5
heartburn once a week or more	22.4
increased stools when pain begins often	13.6
looser stools when pain begins often	17.0
mucus per rectum	6.4
nausea once a month or more	5.8

Symptom	%
pain for greater than 10 years	11.5
pain relieved by defecation often	25.1
pain severity (moderate or worse)	27.8
painful defecation often	11.8
passes greater than 3 times per day	2.5
passes less than or equal to 1 stool per week	2.1
stools loose and watery	12.9
stools often hard	29.7
strain to pass stools often	30.8
takes 3-10 laxatives per week	6.8
urgency often	23.3
uses fingers to facilitate defecation often	23.7
vomiting once a month or more	2.8

wears a pad for fecal incontinence	6.1

Molander, Milson, Ekelund, et al. (1990)
n = 4206
Diagnostic Criteria:
Gender: 0/4206
Age: elderly

Race:
Population Setting: community
Nationality: Sweden
Other Sample Characteristics:
Method of Reporting: postal survey
Timeframe: [1]current; [2]lifetime

Symptom	%
gynecological burning[1]	17.9
gynecological itching[1]	16.7
pain of a gynecological nature[1]	6.7

Symptom	%
urinary incontinence[1]	16.9
urinary incontinence[2]	22.7
vaginal discharge[1]	12.9

Matthews, Wing, Kuller, et al. (1994)
n = 152
Diagnostic Criteria:
Gender: 0/152
Age: 47
Race:

Population Setting: community
Nationality: US
Other Sample Characteristics:
Method of Reporting: self-report
Timeframe: 2 weeks

Symptom	%
aches in neck and/or skull	8
body worry	9
cold sweats	1
constipation	7
crying spells	14
depressed	21
dizzy spells	3
excitable	14

Symptom	%
forgetful	6
headache	22
heart pounding	6
pain	7
rashes	5
trouble sleeping	13

Roberts, Lewinsohn, & Seeley (1995)
n = 1,664
Diagnostic Criteria:
Gender: [1]801/[2]863
Age: seniors in high school
Race:

Population Setting: community
Nationality: US
Other Sample Characteristics:
Method of Reporting: self-report
Timeframe: current

Symptom	%
agitation[1]	1.5
agitation[2]	3.0
anhedonia[1]	2.6
anhedonia[2]	4.8
concentration[1]	5.8
concentration[2]	9.6
decreased appetite[1]	3.1
decreased appetite[2]	7.4
depressed mood[1]	6.0
depressed mood[2]	13.9
excessive guilt[1]	1.6
excessive guilt[2]	3.5
hyperinsomnia[1]	3.1
hyperinsomnia[2]	5.8
increased appetite[1]	1.9
increased appetite[2]	3.0
indecision[1]	2.2
indecision[2]	5.3
initial insomnia[1]	4.6
initial insomnia[2]	8.6
loss of energy[1]	6.2
loss of energy[2]	10.9
middle insomnia[1]	1.4
middle insomnia[2]	4.2
motor disturbance[1]	3.2
motor disturbance[2]	6.5
retardation[1]	2.0
retardation[2]	3.3
sleep disturbance[1]	8.2

Symptom	%
sleep disturbance[2]	15.3
suicidal ideation[1]	0.7
suicidal ideation[2]	1.0
suicide attempt[1]	0.0
suicide attempt[2]	0.1
suicide plan[1]	0.2
suicide plan[2]	0.1
terminal insomnia[1]	1.1
terminal insomnia[2]	2.3
thinking difficulties[1]	7.1
thinking difficulties[2]	12.1
thoughts of death/ suicide[1]	1.6
thoughts of death/ suicide[2]	1.5
thoughts of death[1]	1.5
thoughts of death[2]	1.4
weight gain[1]	0.9
weight gain[2]	2.2
weight loss[1]	1.0
weight loss[2]	4.5
weight/ appetite disturbance[1]	5.3
weight/ appetite disturbance[2]	11.7
worthlessness/ guilt[1]	3.0
worthlessness/ guilt[2]	8.2
worthlessness[1]	2.6
worthlessness[2]	6.0

Neugarte & Kraines (1965)
n = 410
Diagnostic Criteria:
Gender: 0/410
Age: [1]13-18; [2]20-29; [3]30-44; [4]55-64
Race:

Population Setting: community
Nationality: US
Other Sample Characteristics:
Method of Reporting: symptom checklist
Timeframe:

Symptom	%
aches in back of neck and skull[1]	27

Symptom	%
aches in back of neck and skull[2]	26

aches in back of neck and skull[3]	36
aches in back of neck and skull[4]	40
blind spots before the eyes[1]	12
blind spots before the eyes[2]	2
blind spots before the eyes[3]	9
blind spots before the eyes[4]	5
breast pains[1]	20
breast pains[2]	28
breast pains[3]	31
breast pains[4]	6
can't concentrate[1]	65
can't concentrate[2]	52
can't concentrate[3]	56
can't concentrate[4]	15
cold hands and feet[1]	53
cold hands and feet[2]	40
cold hands and feet[3]	36
cold hands and feet[4]	17
cold sweats[1]	19
cold sweats[2]	6
cold sweats[3]	13
cold sweats[4]	4
constipation[1]	28
constipation[2]	50
constipation[3]	36
constipation[4]	31
crying spells[1]	58
crying spells[2]	50
crying spells[3]	36
crying spells[4]	6
diarrhea[1]	29
diarrhea[2]	46
diarrhea[3]	25
diarrhea[4]	31
dizzy spells[1]	39
dizzy spells[2]	30
dizzy spells[3]	36

dizzy spells[4]	26
excitable[1]	68
excitable[2]	64
excitable[3]	51
excitable[4]	20
feel blue and depressed[1]	79
feel blue and depressed[2]	88
feel blue and depressed[3]	62
feel blue and depressed[4]	46
feeling of fright or panic[1]	45
feeling of fright or panic[2]	20
feeling of fright or panic[3]	18
feeling of fright or panic[4]	9
feeling of suffocation[1]	9
feeling of suffocation[2]	0
feeling of suffocation[3]	13
feeling of suffocation[4]	0
flooding[1]	23
flooding[2]	22
flooding[3]	40
flooding[4]	0
forgetfulness[1]	49
forgetfulness[2]	52
forgetfulness[3]	51
forgetfulness[4]	51
headaches[1]	77
headaches[2]	80
headaches[3]	76
headaches[4]	45
hot flushes[1]	29
hot flushes[2]	6
hot flushes[3]	24
hot flushes[4]	40
irritable and nervous[1]	90
irritable and nervous[2]	76
irritable and nervous[3]	82
irritable and nervous[4]	48
numbness and tingling[1]	18
numbness and tingling[2]	14
numbness and tingling[3]	27
numbness and tingling[4]	17
pounding of the heart[1]	29

pounding of the heart[2]	22
pounding of the heart[3]	31
pounding of the heart[4]	32
rheumatic pains[1]	7
rheumatic pains[2]	6
rheumatic pains[3]	33
rheumatic pains[4]	54
skin crawls[1]	11
skin crawls[2]	6
skin crawls[3]	5
skin crawls[4]	6
tired feelings[1]	82
tired feelings[2]	96
tired feelings[3]	84
tired feelings[4]	65
trouble sleeping[1]	49
trouble sleeping[2]	44
trouble sleeping[3]	45

trouble sleeping[4]	58
weight gain[1]	47
weight gain[2]	30
weight gain[3]	40
weight gain[4]	38
worry about body[1]	35
worry about body[2]	20
worry about body[3]	19
worry about body[4]	9
worry about nervous breakdown[1]	10
worry about nervous breakdown[2]	6
worry about nervous breakdown[3]	11
worry about nervous breakdown[4]	5

Neugarte & Kraines (1965)
n = 410
Diagnostic Criteria:
Gender: 0/410
Age: 45-54
Race:
Population Setting: community

Nationality: US
Other Sample Characteristics:
[1]pre/post menopausal; [2]menopausal;
Method of Reporting: symptom
checklist
Timeframe:

Symptom	%
aches in back of neck and skull[2]	46
aches in back of neck and skull[1]	34
aches in back of neck and skull[2]	40
blind spots before the eyes[1]	14
blind spots before the eyes[2]	22
breast pains[1]	10
breast pains[2]	37
can't concentrate[1]	46
can't concentrate[2]	49

Symptom	%
cold hands and feet[2]	42
cold hands and feet[1]	31
cold sweats[1]	16
cold sweats[2]	32
constipation[1]	24
constipation[2]	37
crying spells[1]	38
crying spells[2]	42
diarrhea[1]	20
diarrhea[2]	24
dizzy spells[1]	36
dizzy spells[2]	40
excitable[1]	47

excitable[2]	59
feel blue and depressed[1]	56
feel blue and depressed[2]	78
feeling of fright or panic[1]	22
feeling of fright or panic[2]	22
feeling of suffocation[1]	2
feeling of suffocation[2]	29
flooding[1]	24
flooding[2]	51
forgetfulness[1]	60
forgetfulness[2]	64
headaches[1]	47
headaches[2]	71
hot flushes[1]	28
hot flushes[2]	68
irritable and nervous[1]	71
irritable and nervous[2]	92
numbness and tingling[1]	37

numbness and tingling[2]	37
pounding of the heart[1]	36
pounding of the heart[2]	44
rheumatic pains[1]	46
rheumatic pains[2]	49
skin crawls[1]	3
skin crawls[2]	15
tired feelings[1]	71
tired feelings[2]	88
trouble sleeping[1]	40
trouble sleeping[2]	51
weight gain[1]	41
weight gain[2]	61
worry about body[1]	24
worry about body[2]	24
worry about nervous breakdown[1]	7
worry about nervous breakdown[2]	5

Sternbach (1986)
n = 1,254
Diagnostic Criteria:
Gender: 629/625
Age: 18 and over
Race: 1065/108/81/0/0/0

Population Setting: community
Nationality: US
Other Sample Characteristics:
Method of Reporting: telephone interview
Timeframe: 12 months

Symptom	%
backaches	56
dental pains	27
headaches	73
joint pains	51

Symptom	%
muscle pains	53
premenstrual/menstrual	40
stomach pains	46

McLean, Dikmen, Temkin, et al. (1984)
n = 102
Diagnostic Criteria:
Gender: 65/37
Age: 24.52
Race: 99/0/0/0/0/3

Population Setting: friends of head-injured patients
Nationality: US
Other Sample Characteristics:
Method of Reporting: symptom checklist
Timeframe: current

Symptom	%
anxiety	32
blurred vision	3
concentration	8
difficulties with memory	6
dizziness	13
fatigue	31
headaches	28

Symptom	%
insomnia	18
irritability	34
sensitivity to light	22
sensitivity to noise	13
temper	20

Norton, Harrison, Hauch, et al. (1985)
n = 64
Diagnostic Criteria:
Gender: 14/50
Age: 30.4(8.8); 18-60
Race:

Population Setting: university
extension course students
Nationality: Canada
Other Sample Characteristics:
experienced one or more panic
attacks in last year
Method of Reporting: questionnaire
Timeframe: during panic

Symptom	%
chest pains	46.7
choking	38.6
difficulty breathing	54.8
dizziness	68.8
fainting	62.5
feelings of unreality	54.7

Symptom	%
flushing	69.8
going crazy	60.8
heart pounding	93.8
sweating	90.6
tingling	40.9
trembling	90.5

Heaton, O'Donnell, Braddon, et al. (1992)
n = 1,058
Diagnostic Criteria:
Gender: [1]0/1058
Age: [1]25-29; [2]30-39; [3]40-49; [4]50-59; [5]60-69
Race:

Population Setting: community
Nationality: UK
Other Sample Characteristics:
Method of Reporting: structured
questionnaire
Timeframe: 1 year

Symptom	%
abdominal bloating[1]	14.8
abdominal bloating[2]	9.8
abdominal bloating[3]	17.6
abdominal bloating[4]	20.4
abdominal bloating[5]	16.7
incomplete evacuation[1]	10.2

Symptom	%
incomplete evacuation[2]	12.5
incomplete evacuation[3]	17.1
incomplete evacuation[4]	14.8
incomplete evacuation[5]	16.7
passage of mucus[1]	14.1
passage of mucus[2]	17.7

passage of mucus[3]	16.6
passage of mucus[4]	16.2
passage of mucus[5]	7.1
RAP associated with looser stools[1]	6.2
RAP associated with looser stools[2]	4.9
RAP associated with looser stools[3]	8.5
RAP associated with looser stools[4]	4.9
RAP associated with looser stools[5]	7.1
RAP associated with more frequent defecation[1]	4.9
RAP associated with more frequent defecation[2]	4.0
RAP associated with more frequent defecation[3]	6.0
RAP associated with more frequent defecation[4]	5.6
RAP associated with more frequent defecation[5]	9.5
RAP relieved by defecation[1]	11.8
RAP relieved by defecation[2]	8.2
RAP relieved by defecation[3]	12.1
RAP relieved by defecation[4]	8.5
RAP relieved by defecation[5]	13.1

recurrent abdominal pain (RAP)[1]	25.9
recurrent abdominal pain (RAP)[2]	24.7
recurrent abdominal pain (RAP)[3]	25.1
recurrent abdominal pain (RAP)[4]	22.5
recurrent abdominal pain (RAP)[5]	25.0
straining to finish defecation[1]	2.3
straining to finish defecation[2]	5.5
straining to finish defecation[3]	6.0
straining to finish defecation[4]	7.0
straining to finish defecation[5]	7.1
urgency[1]	9.9
urgency[2]	12.9
urgency[3]	15.4
urgency[4]	16.1
urgency[5]	22.7
watery stools[1]	3.4
watery stools[2]	1.5
watery stools[3]	3.0
watery stools[4]	2.7
watery stools[5]	1.5

Heaton, O'Donnell, Braddon, et al. (1992)
n = 838
Diagnostic Criteria:
Gender: 838/0
Age: [1]40-49; [2]50-59; [3]60-69
Race:

Population Setting: community
Nationality: UK
Other Sample Characteristics:
Method of Reporting: structured questionnaire
Timeframe: 1 year

Symptom	%
abdominal bloating[1]	6.3
abdominal bloating[2]	3.5
abdominal bloating[3]	8.2
incomplete evacuation[1]	6.5
incomplete evacuation[2]	4.0
incomplete evacuation[3]	3.9
passage of mucus[1]	5.6
passage of mucus[2]	6.2
passage of mucus[3]	2.2
RAP associated with looser stools[1]	4.0
RAP associated with looser stools[2]	1.8
RAP associated with looser stools[3]	2.8
RAP associated with more frequent defecation[1]	2.8
RAP associated with more frequent defecation[2]	1.3
RAP associated with more frequent defecation[3]	2.2
RAP relieved by defecation[1]	7.0

Symptom	%
RAP relieved by defecation[2]	4.0
RAP relieved by defecation[3]	5.0
recurrent abdominal pain (RAP)[1]	15.4
recurrent abdominal pain (RAP)[2]	17.7
recurrent abdominal pain (RAP)[3]	15.4
straining to finish defecation[1]	2.1
straining to finish defecation[2]	1.8
straining to finish defecation[3]	1.6
urgency[1]	6.1
urgency[2]	7.6
urgency[3]	14.0
watery stools[1]	3.8
watery stools[2]	1.6
watery stools[3]	4.0

Lee & Rittenhouse (1991)
n = 594
Diagnostic Criteria:
Gender: 0/594
Age: 33.4(7.24); 21-50
Race: 508/9/15/54/0/6

Population Setting: registered nurses
Nationality: US
Other Sample Characteristics: during perimenstrual period
Method of Reporting: postal survey
Timeframe:

Symptom	%
anxious, tense, irritable	62.5
backache	44.8
constipation	22.1
cramps	55.6
depression, crying	35.8
diarrhea	22.0
fatigue	54.6

Symptom	%
food cravings	50.3
headache	34.9
mood swings	52.8
painful breasts	53.8
skin disorders	24.3
weight gain, swelling	66.3

Lee & Rittenhouse (1991)
n = 760
Diagnostic Criteria:
Gender: 0/760
Age: [1]21-25; [2]26-30; [3]31-35; [4]36-40;
[5]41-45; [6]46-50
Race:

Population Setting: registered nurses
Nationality: US
Other Sample Characteristics: during
perimenstrual phase
Method of Reporting: postal survey
Timeframe:

Symptom	%
anxious, tense, irritable[1]	71.8
anxious, tense, irritable[2]	51.3
anxious, tense, irritable[3]	65.8
anxious, tense, irritable[4]	57.9
anxious, tense, irritable[5]	60.3
anxious, tense, irritable[6]	50.0
backache[1]	53.6
backache[2]	43.4
backache[3]	45.8
backache[4]	37.7
backache[5]	43.9
backache[6]	50
constipation[1]	24.5
constipation[2]	23.5
constipation[3]	24.5
constipation[4]	18.8
constipation[5]	18.3
constipation[6]	26.3
cramps[1]	61.9
cramps[2]	69.6
cramps[3]	51.6
cramps[4]	50.2
cramps[5]	45.2
cramps[6]	50
depression, crying[1]	47.3
depression, crying[2]	37.8
depression, crying[3]	37.2
depression, crying[4]	52.4
depression, crying[5]	24.7
depression, crying[6]	15.8
diarrhea[1]	22.1

Symptom	%
diarrhea[2]	27.4
diarrhea[3]	24.7
diarrhea[4]	23.8
diarrhea[5]	15.5
diarrhea[6]	7.9
fatigue[1]	65.5
fatigue[2]	54.7
fatigue[3]	57.2
fatigue[4]	49.2
fatigue[5]	46.6
fatigue[6]	52.6
food cravings[1]	61.8
food cravings[2]	51
food cravings[3]	49
food cravings[4]	49.2
food cravings[5]	41.6
food cravings[6]	44.7
headache[1]	35.4
headache[2]	35.9
headache[3]	35.3
headache[4]	28.7
headache[5]	46.6
headache[6]	34.2
mood swings[1]	60
mood swings[2]	60.3
mood swings[3]	52.3
mood swings[4]	52.4
mood swings[5]	43.8
mood swings[6]	37.8
painful breasts[1]	60.9
painful breasts[2]	53.8

painful breasts[3]	52.3
painful breasts[4]	51.6
painful breasts[5]	54.8
painful breasts[6]	52.6
skin disorders[1]	36.4
skin disorders[2]	31.1
skin disorders[3]	26.8
skin disorders[4]	16.4

skin disorders[5]	12.3
skin disorders[6]	10.5
weight gain, swelling[1]	70
weight gain, swelling[2]	69.8
weight gain, swelling[3]	67.3
weight gain, swelling[4]	60.4
weight gain, swelling[5]	67.1
weight gain, swelling[6]	65.8

Cuijpers, Wesseling, Swaen, et al. (1994)
n = 482
Diagnostic Criteria:
Gender: 226/256
Age: 6-12
Race:

Population Setting: primary school
Nationality: Netherlands
Other Sample Characteristics:
Method of Reporting: postal survey; parent report
Timeframe: [1]lifetime; [2]1 year

Symptom	%
attacks of shortness of breath with wheeze[1]	19
attacks of shortness of breath with wheeze[2]	10
chronic cough[1]	13
exercise-induced shortness of breath[1]	15

Symptom	%
exercise-induced shortness of breath[2]	12
wheeze[1]	29
wheeze[2]	15

Cuijpers, Wesseling, Swaen, et al. (1994)
n = 482
Diagnostic Criteria: doctor-diagnosed
Gender: [1]226/[2]256
Age:
Race:

Population Setting: primary school
Nationality: Netherlands
Other Sample Characteristics:
Method of Reporting: postal survey; parent report
Timeframe: lifetime

Symptom	%
chronic cough[1]	15.0
chronic cough[2]	11.3

Cuijpers, Wesseling, Swaen, et al. (1994)

n = 482
Diagnostic Criteria: doctor-diagnosed

Gender: [1]226/[2]256
Age:
Race:
Population Setting: primary school
Nationality: Netherlands

Other Sample Characteristics:
Method of Reporting: postal survey;
parent report
Timeframe: 1 year

Symptom	%
attacks, shortness of breath, & wheeze previous year[1]	12.4
attacks, shortness of breath, & wheeze previous year[2]	7.0
shortness of breath previous year[1]	15.9

Symptom	%
shortness of breath previous year[2]	9.0
wheeze previous year[1]	15.5
wheeze previous year[2]	14.5

Cuijpers, Wesseling, Swaen, et al. (1994)
n = 482
Diagnostic Criteria: doctor-diagnosed
Gender:
Age: [1]6-9; [2]10-12
Race:

Population Setting: primary school
Nationality: Netherlands
Other Sample Characteristics:
Method of Reporting: postal survey;
parent report
Timeframe: lifetime

Symptom	%
chronic cough[1]	14.9
chronic cough[2]	10.2

Cuijpers, Wesseling, Swaen, et al. (1994)
n = 482
Diagnostic Criteria: doctor-diagnosed
Gender:
Age: [1]6-9; [2]10-12
Race:

Population Setting: primary school
Nationality: Netherlands
Other Sample Characteristics:
Method of Reporting: postal survey;
parent report
Timeframe: 1 year

Symptom	%
attacks, shortness of breath, & wheeze previous year[1]	10.2

Symptom	%
attacks, shortness of breath, & wheeze previous year[2]	8.6

shortness of breath previous year[1]	11.9
shortness of breath previous year[2]	12.8

wheeze previous year[1]	14.2
wheeze previous year[2]	16

Larsson, Lundback, & Jonsson (1997)
n = 529
Diagnostic Criteria:
Gender: 342/187
Age:
Race:

Population Setting: community
Nationality: Sweden
Other Sample Characteristics:
Method of Reporting: postal survey
Timeframe:

Symptom	%
apnoeas	8.3
apnoeas, not rested, & nodding off	0.8
attacks of breathlessness	8.1
long-standing cough	13.4
nodding off	7.0
not rested	27.6
recurrent wheeze	9.8
snoring	11.7

Symptom	%
snoring, apnoeas, & nodding off	1.3
snoring, not rested, & nodding off	1.3
snoring, apnoeas, & not rested	2.5
snoring, apnoeas, not rested, & nodding off	0.8
sputum production	17.8

Larsson, Lundback, & Jonsson (1997)
n = 529
Diagnostic Criteria:
Gender: [1]342/[2]187
Age:
Race:

Population Setting: community
Nationality: Sweden
Other Sample Characteristics:
Method of Reporting: postal survey
Timeframe:

Symptom	%
apnoeas[1]	10.8
apnoeas[2]	3.7
attacks of breathlessness[1]	8.2
attacks of breathlessness[2]	8.0
long-standing cough[1]	10.5
long-standing cough[2]	18.7
nodding off[1]	8.5
nodding off[2]	4.3

Symptom	%
not rested[1]	27.5
not rested[2]	27.8
recurrent wheeze[1]	10.8
recurrent wheeze[2]	8.0
snoring[1]	13.7
snoring[2]	8.0
sputum production[1]	19.3
sputum production[2]	15.0

Larsson, Lundback, & Jonsson (1997)
n = 119
Diagnostic Criteria:
Gender: [1]75/[2]44
Age: 41-42
Race:

Population Setting: community
Nationality: Sweden
Other Sample Characteristics:
Method of Reporting: postal survey
Timeframe:

Symptom	%
apnoeas[1]	9.3
apnoeas[2]	6.8
nodding off[1]	5.3
nodding off[2]	4.5

Symptom	%
not rested[1]	32.0
not rested[2]	25.0
snoring[1]	10.7

Larsson, Lundback, & Jonsson (1997)
n = 171
Diagnostic Criteria:
Gender: [1]114/[2]57
Age: 56-57
Race:

Population Setting: community
Nationality: Sweden
Other Sample Characteristics:
Method of Reporting: postal survey
Timeframe:

Symptom	%
apnoeas[1]	14.9
apnoeas[2]	3.5
nodding off[1]	11.4
nodding off[2]	3.5

Symptom	%
not rested[1]	33.3
not rested[2]	35.1
snoring[1]	23.7
snoring[2]	3.5

Larsson, Lundback, & Jonsson (1997)
n = 239
Diagnostic Criteria:
Gender: [1]153/[2]86
Age: 71-72
Race:

Population Setting: community
Nationality: Sweden
Other Sample Characteristics:
Method of Reporting: postal survey
Timeframe:

Symptom	%
apnoeas[1]	8.5
apnoeas[2]	2.3
nodding off[1]	7.8
nodding off[2]	4.7

Symptom	%
not rested[1]	20.9
not rested[2]	24.4
snoring[1]	7.8
snoring[2]	10.5

Svensson, Anderson, Hagstad, et al.
(1989)
n = 1,218

Diagnostic Criteria:
Gender: 0/1,218
Age: 38-64

Race:
Population Setting: community
Nationality: Sweden

Symptom	%
low-back pain	15.8

Other Sample Characteristics:
Method of Reporting: postal survey
Timeframe: lifetime

Svensson, Anderson, Hagstad, et al.
(1989)
$\underline{n}$ = 1,218
Diagnostic Criteria:
Gender: 0/1,218
Age: [1]38-49; [2]50-64

Race:
Population Setting: community
Nationality: Sweden
Other Sample Characteristics:
Method of Reporting: postal survey
Timeframe: [1]lifetime

Symptom	%
low-back pain[1]	66.7
low-back pain[2]	65.6

Svensson, Anderson, Hagstad, et al.
(1989)
$\underline{n}$ = 1,218
Diagnostic Criteria:
Gender: 0/1,218
Age: [1]38-49; [2]50-64

Race:
Population Setting: community
Nationality: Sweden
Other Sample Characteristics:
Method of Reporting: postal survey
Timeframe: 1 month

Symptom	%
low-back pain[1]	33.2
low-back pain[2]	36.9

Rasmussen & Olessen (1992)
$\underline{n}$ = 740
Diagnostic Criteria: operational
diagnostic criteria of the HIS
Gender: 387/353
Age:
Race:

Population Setting: community
Nationality: Denmark
Other Sample Characteristics:
Method of Reporting: structured
interview
Timeframe: lifetime

Symptom	%
benign cough headache	1

Symptom	%
benign exertional	1

headache	
chronic tension-type headache	3
cold stimulus headache	15
episodic tension-type headache	66
external compression headache	4

fever headache	63
hangover	72
headache associated with sexual activity	1
idiopathic stabbing headache	2
migraine with aura	6
migraine without aura	9

Rasmussen & Olessen (1992)
n = 740
Diagnostic Criteria: operational diagnostic criteria of the HIS
Gender: [1]387/[2]353
Age:
Race:

Population Setting: community
Nationality: Denmark
Other Sample Characteristics:
Method of Reporting: structured interview
Timeframe: lifetime

Symptom	%
cold stimulus hangover[1]	12
cold stimulus hangover[2]	17
external compression headache[1]	2
external compression headache[2]	6
fever headache[1]	57

Symptom	%
fever headache[2]	69
hangover[1]	75
hangover[2]	67
idiopathic stabbing headache[1]	2
idiopathic stabbing headache[2]	3

Sternfeld, Stang, & Sidney (1995)
n = 74,962
Diagnostic Criteria:
Gender:
Age: [1]44.1 (14.7); [2]44.0 (13.7); [3]39.9 (13.1); [4]40.1 (13.4)
Race: [1]17381/4084/0/951/0/789; [2]15955/3241/0/920/0/795;

[3]10996/3403/0/835/0/819;
[4]10591/2663/0/799/0/754
Population Setting: HMO enrollees
Nationality: US
Other Sample Characteristics:
Method of Reporting: structured interview
Timeframe: 1 year

Symptom	%
chest pain[1]	13.4
chest pain[2]	12.5

Symptom	%
chest pain[3]	13.1
chest pain[4]	14.6

Rasmussen, Jenson, Schroll, et al.
(1992)
n = 740
Diagnostic Criteria: structured
diagnostic headache interview
Gender: 387/353
Age: 25-64

Race:
Population Setting: community
Nationality: Denmark
Other Sample Characteristics:
Method of Reporting: structured
interview and examination
Timeframe: 1 year

Symptom	%
chronic tension-type	3
coexisting migraine and tension-type	9
episodic tension-type	63
migraine with aura	4
migraine with aura and tension-type	3
migraine without aura	6

Symptom	%
migraine without aura and tension-type	5
migraine, total	10
migrainous disorder and tension-type	1
migrainous disorders	1
tension-type, total	74
tension-type-like	8

Rasmussen, Jenson, Schroll, et al.
(1992)
n = 740
Diagnostic Criteria: structured
diagnostic headache interview
Gender: [1]387/[2]353
Age: 25-64

Race:
Population Setting: community
Nationality: Denmark
Other Sample Characteristics:
Method of Reporting: structured
interview and examination
Timeframe: 1 year

Symptom	%
chronic tension-type[1]	2
chronic tension-type[2]	5
coexisting migraine and tension-type[1]	4
coexisting migraine and tension-type[2]	4
episodic tension-type[1]	56
episodic tension-type[2]	71
migraine with aura and tension type[1]	2
migraine with aura and tension type[2]	4
migraine with aura[1]	3
migraine with aura[2]	5

Symptom	%
migraine without aura and tension-type[1]	2
migraine without aura and tension-type[2]	9
migraine without aura[1]	2
migraine without aura[2]	11
migraine, total[1]	6
migraine, total[2]	15
migrainous disorder and tension-type[1]	1
migrainous disorder and tension-type[2]	1
migrainous disorder[1]s	2
migrainous disorder[2]s	1

tension-type total[2]	86
tension-type, total[1]	63

tension-type-like[1]	5
tension-type-like[2]	11

Saykin, Janssen, & Sprehn (1991)
n = 21
Diagnostic Criteria: structured
diagnostic headache interview
Gender: 21/0
Age: 31.45 (5.53)
Race:

Population Setting: community
Nationality: US
Other Sample Characteristics:
[1]baseline; [2]18 months
Method of Reporting: neurological
examination
Timeframe: current

Symptom	%
concentration[1]	0
concentration[2]	0
depression[1]	5
depression[2]	10
headache[1]	0
headache[2]	5
irritability[1]	0
irritability[2]	5

Symptom	%
memory[1]	10
memory[2]	5
paresthesia[1]	0
paresthesia[2]	0
speech[1]	14
speech[2]	5
weakness[1]	0
weakness[2]	0

Kroenke & Price (1993)
n = 13,538
Diagnostic Criteria:
Gender: 6,498/7,040
Age: 18+
Race: 10736/0/0/0/0/0

Population Setting: community
Nationality: US
Other Sample Characteristics:
Method of Reporting: structured
interview
Timeframe: lifetime

Symptom	%
abdominal pain	24.0
abdominal pain	58.3
arm or leg pain	25.1
back pain	31.1
chest pain	25.2
constipation	16.7
diarrhea	12.2
dizziness	24.3
dyspnea	15.0
dysuria	18.3
fainting	11.4

Symptom	%
fatigue	21.8
gas or bloating	20.6
headache	25.9
heavy menses	13.1
insomnia	19.6
irregular menses	14.7
joint pain	38.3
loss of feeling	8.2
missed menses	6.4
nausea	15.0
painful menses	17.7

palpitations	18.1
trouble walking	20.2
vision blurred	17.3

vomiting	6.7
weakness	11.8

Kroenke & Price (1993)
n = 7094
Diagnostic Criteria:
Gender: 0/7094
Age: 18+
Race:

Population Setting: community
Nationality: US
Other Sample Characteristics:
Method of Reporting: structured
interview
Timeframe: lifetime

Symptom	%
abdominal pain	58.3
arm or leg pain	55.4
back pain	55.9
blurred vision	54.5
chest pain	50.8
constipation	77.9
diarrhea	58.3
dizziness	63.9
dyspnea	58.3
dysuria	68.0
fainting	68.1

Symptoms	%
fatigue	65.8
gas or bloating	62.3
headache	67.7
insomnia	60.7
joint pain	53.3
loss of feeling	55.2
nausea	69.1
palpitations	63.4
vomiting	64.2
walking trouble	50.9
weakness	57.5

Kroenke & Price (1993)
n = 10,737
Diagnostic Criteria:
Gender:
Age: 18+
Race: 10,737/0/0/0/0/0

Population Setting: community
Nationality: US
Other Sample Characteristics:
Method of Reporting: structured
interview
Timeframe: lifetime

Symptom	%
abdominal pain	81.1
arm or leg pain	80.1
back pain	82.6
blurred vision	80.9
chest pain	79.7
constipation	79.6
diarrhea	83.9

Symptom	%
dizziness	80.2
dyspnea	79.2
dysuria	84.4
fainting	84.4
fatigue	84.0
gas or bloating	78.4
headache	78.2

heavy menses	82.3
insomnia	81.2
irregular menses	80.8
joint pain	80.0
loss of feeling	83.9
missed menses	83.8

nausea	77.6
painful menses	80.4
palpitations	84.5
vomiting	79.4
walking trouble	81.0
weakness	81.0

Breslau, Roth, & Rosenthal (1996)
n = 1,007
Diagnostic Criteria:
Gender: 386/621
Age: 26; 21-30
Race: 813/194/0/0/0/0

Population Setting: HMO members
Nationality: US
Other Sample Characteristics:
Method of Reporting: structured
interview
Timeframe: lifetime

Symptom	%
hypersomnia alone	8.2
insomnia alone	16.6

Symptom	%
insomnia and hypersomnia	8.0

Breslau, Roth, & Rosenthal (1996)
n = 1,007
Diagnostic Criteria:
Gender: [1]388/ [2]619
Age:
Race: Population Setting: HMO
members

Nationality: US
Other Sample Characteristics:
Method of Reporting: structured
interview
Timeframe: lifetime

Symptom	%
hypersomnia alone[1]	9.3
hypersomnia alone[2]	7.6
insomnia alone[1]	16.0

Symptom	%
insomnia alone[2]	17.0
insomnia and hypersomnia[1]	5.4
insomnia and hypersomnia[2]	9.7

Breslau, Roth, & Rosenthal (1996)
n = 1,007
Diagnostic Criteria:
Gender:
Age:
Race: [1]0/194/0/0/0/0; [2]813/0/0/0/0/0

Population Setting: HMO members
Nationality: US
Other Sample Characteristics:
Method of Reporting: structured
interview
Timeframe: lifetime

Symptom	%
hypersomnia alone[1]	7.7
hypersomnia alone[2]	8.4
insomnia alone[1]	13.9
insomnia alone[2]	17.2

Symptom	%
insomnia and hypersomnia[1]	5.7
insomnia and hypersomnia[2]	8.6

Menza & Rosen (1995)
n = 47
Diagnostic Criteria:
Gender: 25/22
Age: 61 (15.3)
Race:

Population Setting: family of
Parkinson's patients
Nationality: US
Other Sample Characteristics:
Method of Reporting: self-report
Timeframe:

Symptom	%
anxiety	17
bed-wetting	3
depression	6
difficulty breathing at night	11

Symptoms	%
jerks and twitches at night at night	8
morning headaches	22
restless legs	14
snoring at night	64

Albert & Beck (1975)
n = 63
Diagnostic Criteria:
Gender: 36/27
Age: 11-15
Race: 62/0/0/1/0/0

Population Setting: parochial school
students
Nationality: US
Other Sample Characteristics:
Method of Reporting: self-report
Timeframe: current

Symptom	%
suicidal ideation	35

Lavie (1981)
n = 1,502
Diagnostic Criteria:
Gender: 1,262/240
Age:
Race:
Population Setting: industrial workers

Nationality: Israel
Other Sample Characteristics: [1]while
falling asleep; [2]while sleeping;
[3]awakening
Method of Reporting: structured
interview
Timeframe:

Symptom	%
difficulties breathing and suffocating[3]	3.0

Symptom	%
difficulty breathing and suffocation[1]	5.8

disorientation[1]	1.6
disorientation[3]	1.0
excessive leg movements[2]	9.6
excessive movements in sleep[2]	33.2
feelings of worry and tension[1]	12.0
headaches[1]	7.2
headaches[3]	5.5
midsleep awakening[3]	17.0
pain in different parts of	7.5

the body[1]	
pain in different parts of the body[3]	4.7
paralysis of the legs[1]	0.7
paralysis of the legs[3]	0.5
sleep walking[2]	0.4
snoring[2]	18.5
sweating and feeling hot[1]	7.5
sweating and feeling hot[3]	4.3
talking in one's sleep[2]	3.6
worries and tension[3]	1.4

Lavie (1981)
n = 1,502
Diagnostic Criteria:
Gender: [1]1262/[2]240
Age:
Race:

Population Setting: industrial workers
Nationality: Israel
Other Sample Characteristics:
Method of Reporting: structured interview
Timeframe:

Symptom	%
difficulties falling asleep[1]	6.6
midsleep awakening[1]	10.8
excessive daytime somnolence (EDS)[1]	5.0
difficulties falling asleep and midsleep awakenings[1]	2.7
EDS and difficulties falling asleep and midsleep awakening[1]	3.1

Symptom	%
difficulties falling asleep[2]	12.1
midsleep awakenings[2]	12.1
excessive daytime somnolence[2]	4.6
difficulties falling asleep and midsleep awakenings[2]	7.1
EDS and difficulties falling asleep and midsleep awakenings[2]	2.1

Droller & Pemberton (1953)
n = 476
Diagnostic Criteria:
Gender: [1]192/[2]284
Age: [1]67+; [2]62+
Race:

Population Setting: community
Nationality: UK
Other Sample Characteristics:
Method of Reporting: medical exam
Timeframe:

Symptom	%
vertigo[1]	27.6

vertigo[2]	53.9

Enright, Kronmal, Higgins, et al.
(1994)
n = 2,359
Diagnostic Criteria:
Gender: [1]716/[2]1,643
Age: 65+
Race:

Population Setting: community
Nationality: US
Other Sample Characteristics: non-smokers
Method of Reporting: structured interview
Timeframe:

Symptom	%
cough > 3 months[1]	5.7
cough > 3 months[2]	7.4
cough day and night[1]	5.7
cough day and night[2]	9.1
frequent cough[1]	6.1
frequent cough[2]	8.2
frequent phlegm[1]	12.5
frequent phlegm[2]	8.0
grade 3 dyspnea[1]	10.0

Symptom	%
grade 3 dyspnea[2]	6.4
phlegm > 3 months[1]	11.5
phlegm > 3 months[2]	7.9
phlegm day and night[1]	11.4
phlegm day and night[2]	7.4
wheeze and dyspnea[1]	6.0
wheeze and dyspnea[2]	6.9
wheeze day and night[1]	3.2
wheeze day and night[2]	4.1

Enright, Kronmal, Higgins, et al.
(1994)
n = 2,147
Diagnostic Criteria:
Gender: [1]1,272/[2]875
Age: 65+
Race:

Population Setting: community
Nationality: US
Other Sample Characteristics: former smokers
Method of Reporting: structured interview
Timeframe:

Symptom	%
cough > 3 months[1]	7.6
cough > 3 months[2]	7.5
cough day and night[1]	8.1
cough day and night[2]	8.6
dyspnea grade 3[1]	9.6
dyspnea grade 3[2]	12.5
frequent cough[1]	7.6
frequent cough[2]	8.6
frequent phlegm[1]	15.4

Symptom	%
frequent phlegm[2]	10.3
phlegm > 3 months[1]	16.0
phlegm > 3 months[2]	9.9
phlegm day and night[1]	14.5
phlegm day and night[2]	8.6
wheeze and dyspnea[1]	7.2
wheeze and dyspnea[2]	9.8
wheeze day and night[1]	5.7
wheeze day and night[2]	4.5

Enright, Kronmal, Higgins, et al.
(1994)
n = 613
Diagnostic Criteria:
Gender: [1]231/[2]382
Age: 65+
Race:

Population Setting: community
Nationality: US
Other Sample Characteristics: current
smokers
Method of Reporting: structured
interview
Timeframe:

Symptom	%
cough > 3 months[1]	9.2
cough > 3 months[2]	22.8
cough day and night[1]	10.5
cough day and night[2]	24.3
dyspnea grade 3[1]	10.1
dyspnea grade 3[2]	11.5
frequent cough[1]	10.0
frequent cough[2]	25.1
frequent phlegm[1]	13.8

Symptom	%
frequent phlegm[2]	27.7
phlegm > 3 months[1]	13.1
phlegm > 3 months[2]	23.8
phlegm day and night[1]	12.4
phlegm day and night[2]	25.1
wheeze and dyspnea[1]	7.7
wheeze and dyspnea[2]	10.2
wheeze day and night[1]	5.6
wheeze day and night[2]	10.7

Katona, Livingston, Manela, et al.
(1997)
n = 700
Diagnostic Criteria:
Gender: 253/447
Age: 65+
Race:

Population Setting: community
Nationality: UK
Other Sample Characteristics:
Method of Reporting: semi-structured
interview
Timeframe:

Symptom	%
difficulty falling asleep	21
difficulty with light housework	14
does not get out as often as needs to	21
embarrassed by memory problems	13
faintness on rapid rising	11
feeling dizzy	21
feeling weak	12
forgets where put things	26
health getting worse	9

Symptom	%
health limiting mobility	24
health limiting other activities	17
health limiting socializing	7
health problems interfering with desired activity	50
interrupted sleep	33
making effort to remember things	14
not eating well	7

Symptom	%
subjective memory difficulty	34

Newland, Illis, Robinson, et al. (1978)
n = 938
Diagnostic Criteria:
Gender: [1]46/0; [2]233/0; [3]320/0; [4]284/0; [5]55/0
Age: [1]18-20; [2]21-34; [3]35-54; [4]55-74; [5]75+

Race:
Population Setting: community
Nationality: UK
Other Sample Characteristics:
Method of Reporting: postal survey
Timeframe: 1 year

Symptom	%
blind areas before headache[1]	2
blind areas before headache[2]	8
blind areas before headache[3]	21
blind areas before headache[4]	16
blind areas before headache[5]	2
changes in mood before headache[1]	14
changes in mood before headache[2]	47
changes in mood before headache[3]	53
changes in mood before headache[4]	35
changes in mood before headache[5]	3
headache[1]	87
headache[2]	80
headache[3]	56
headache[4]	88
headache[5]	46
pins and needles before headache[1]	0
pins and needles before headache[2]	7

Symptom	%
pins and needles before headache[3]	8
pins and needles before headache[4]	8
pins and needles before headache[5]	1
sickness before headache[1]	7
sickness before headache[2]	36
sickness before headache[3]	64
sickness before headache[4]	20
sickness before headache[5]	3
watery eyes before headache[1]	6
watery eyes before headache[2]	38
watery eyes before headache[3]	45
watery eyes before headache[4]	32
watery eyes before headache[5]	8
zigzag flashes before headache[1]	1
zigzag flashes before headache[2]	10
zigzag flashes before headache[3]	21
zigzag flashes before headache[4]	15

zigzag flashes before headache[5]	1

Newland, Illis, Robinson, et al.
(1978)
n = 938
Diagnostic Criteria:
Gender: [1]0/63; [2]0/276; [3]0/314; [4]0/363; [5]0/110
Age: [1]18-20; [2]21-34; [3]35-54; [4]55-74; [5]75+

Race:
Population Setting: community
Nationality: UK
Other Sample Characteristics:
Method of Reporting: postal survey
Timeframe: 1 year

Symptom	%
blind areas before headache[1]	2.0
blind areas before headache[2]	13.0
blind areas before headache[3]	24.0
blind areas before headache[4]	15.0
blind areas before headache[5]	6.0
changes in mood before headache[1]	17.0
changes in mood before headache[2]	86.0
changes in mood before headache[3]	93.0
changes in mood before headache[4]	63.0
changes in mood before headache[5]	6.0
headache[1]	93.7
headache[2]	96.7
headache[3]	91.1
headache[4]	68.0
headache[5]	52.7
pins and needles before headache[1]	0.0
pins and needles before headache[2]	14.0

Symptom	%
pins and needles before headache[3]	13.0
pins and needles before headache[4]	24.0
pins and needles before headache[5]	2.0
sickness before headache[1]	11.0
sickness before headache[2]	87.0
sickness before headache[3]	96.0
sickness before headache[4]	63.0
sickness before headache[5]	9.0
watery eyes before headache[1]	14.0
watery eyes before headache[2]	84.0
watery eyes before headache[3]	56.0
watery eyes before headache[4]	58.0
watery eyes before headache[5]	18.0
zigzag flashes before headache[1]	3.0
zigzag flashes before headache[2]	23.0
zigzag flashes before headache[3]	24.0
zigzag flashes before headache[4]	38.0

zigzag flashes before headache[5]	7.0

Clifford, Radford, Howell, et al.
(1989)
$\underline{n} = 628$
Diagnostic Criteria:
Gender: 0/628
Age: 7
Race:
Population Setting: school children

Nationality: UK
Other Sample Characteristics:
Method of Reporting: parental
questionnaire
Timeframe: [1]lifetime; [2]past 12
months; [3]12 months

Symptom	%
chest discomfort[3]	7.9
chesty at night[3]	18.2
cough-current[3]	27.9
morning cough[3]	18.5
morning shortness of breath[2]	1.6
morning wheeze[2]	3.5
nocturnal cough[3]	17.3

Symptom	%
nocturnal shortness of breath[2]	1.9
nocturnal wheeze[2]	6.3
shortness of breath[1]	7.2
shortness of breath[2]	4.8
wheeze[1]	15.9
wheeze[2]	9.5

Clifford, Radford, Howell, et al.
(1989)
$\underline{n} = 647$
Diagnostic Criteria:
Gender: 647/0
Age: 7
Race:
Population Setting: school children

Nationality: UK
Other Sample Characteristics:
Method of Reporting: parental
questionnaire
Timeframe: [1]lifetime; [2]past 12
months; [3]12 months

Symptom	%
chest discomfort[3]	13.0
chesty at night[3]	20.3
cough-current[3]	33.7
morning cough[3]	22.6
morning shortness of breath[2]	4.3
morning wheeze[2]	8.9
nocturnal cough[3]	18.2

Symptom	%
nocturnal shortness of breath[2]	5.2
nocturnal wheeze[2]	7.9
shortness of breath[1]	12.3
shortness of breath[2]	9.0
wheeze[1]	22.7
wheeze[2]	14.3

Clifford, Radford, Howell, et al.
(1989)
n = 600
Diagnostic Criteria:
Gender: 0/600
Age: 11
Race:
Population Setting: school children

Nationality: UK
Other Sample Characteristics:
Method of Reporting: parental
questionnaire
Timeframe: [1]lifetime; [2]past 12
months; [3]12 months

Symptom	%
wheeze[1]	16.7
wheeze[2]	10.9
nocturnal wheeze[2]	6.6
morning wheeze[2]	7.3
shortness of breath[1]	13.4
shortness of breath[2]	10.3
nocturnal shortness of breath[2]	10.3

Symptom	%
morning shortness of breath[2]	2.5
cough- current[3]	19.3
nocturnal cough[3]	8.7
morning cough[3]	13.0
chest discomfort[3]	14.2
chesty at night[3]	12.4

Clifford, Radford, Howell, et al.
(1989)
n = 618
Diagnostic Criteria:
Gender: 618/0
Age: 11
Race:
Population Setting: school children

Nationality: UK
Other Sample Characteristics:
Method of Reporting: parental
questionnaire
Timeframe: [1]lifetime; [2]past 12
months; [3]12 months

Symptom	%
wheeze[1]	19.9
wheeze[2]	13.7
nocturnal wheeze[2]	9.1
morning wheeze[2]	8.0
shortness of breath[1]	13.6
shortness of breath[2]	10.0
nocturnal shortness of breath[2]	4.9

Symptom	%
morning shortness of breath[2]	4.1
cough- current[3]	22.2
nocturnal cough[3]	12.4
morning cough[3]	13.8
chest discomfort[3]	15.1

Grant, Atkinson, Hesselink, et al.
(1987)

n = 11
Diagnostic Criteria:

Gender:
Age: 39.3 (11.0)
Race:
Population Setting: community
Nationality: US

Other Sample Characteristics:
homosexual men
Method of Reporting:
neuropsychological testing
Timeframe: current

Symptom	%
neuropsychological abnormality	9

Grant, Atkinson, Hesselink, et al.
(1987)
n = 620
Diagnostic Criteria:
Gender:
Age: 17-26
Race:

Population Setting: college
undergraduates
Nationality: US
Other Sample Characteristics: survey
1
Method of Reporting: self-report
Timeframe: current

Symptom	%	Symptom	%
angry sleep	1.3	memory gaps	9.7
automatic driving	6.7	mental decline	14.5
confusional spells	10.0	olfactory illusions	11.5
deja vu	31.6	panic spells	10.3
discontinuous viewing	3.9	severe headaches	6.9
dysphoric spells	18.4	speaking jargon	23.5
environmental distortion	10.7	speech problems	16.8
episodic numbness	9.4	staring spells	23.2
episodic tinnitus	31.4	suicidal ideation	3.1
gustatory illusions	8.9	temper outbursts	10.3
haptic illusions	16.1	unrecalled anger	1.3
illusion of movement	22.2	unrecalled behaviors	9.4
irresistible sleepiness	18.0	visual fixation	20.7
jamais vu	11.0	visual illusions	12.0
loss of consciousness	2.3	word-finding lapses	26.5

Grant, Atkinson, Hesselink, et al.
(1987)
n = 620
Diagnostic Criteria:
Gender:
Age: 17-27

Race:
Population Setting: college
undergraduates
Nationality: US
Other Sample Characteristics: survey
2

Method of Reporting: self-report   Timeframe: current

Symptom	%
angry sleep	0.3
automatic driving	6.7
cephalic pain	10.5
confusional spells	10.9
deja vu	44.2
discontinuous tv viewing	7.0
dysphoric spells	15.3
environmental distortion	13.9
episodic numbness	10.5
episodic tinnitus	31.1
gustatory illusions	21.0
haptic illusions	28.9
illusion of movement	35.5
irresistible sleepiness	17.1
jamais vu	8.8
loss of consciousness	1.8
memory gaps	11.4
mental decline	5.3

Symptom	%
mice running	4.7
nightmares	3.5
nocturnal sweating	4.7
olfactory illusions	12.6
panic spells	11.3
severe headaches	3.9
speaking jargon	28.9
speech problems	17.0
staring spells	25.4
suicidal ideation	1.8
telephone ringing	1.3
temper outbursts	9.0
unrecalled anger	0.3
unrecalled behaviors	7.5
urinary urgency	8.7
visual fixation	23.6
visual illusions	12.7
word-finding lapses	30.7

Fitzpatrick, Martin, Fossey, et al.
(1993)
n = 1,478
Diagnostic Criteria:
Gender:
Age: 45 (18)

Race:
Population Setting: community
Nationality: UK
Other Sample Characteristics:
Method of Reporting: postal survey
Timeframe: current

Symptom	%
snored at least four nights per week	0.1
snoring occasionally	0.4

Aldrich & Chauncey (1990)
n = 130
Diagnostic Criteria:
Gender:
Age:
Race:

Population Setting: community
Nationality: US
Other Sample Characteristics:
Method of Reporting: postal survey
Timeframe: current

Symptom	%
morning headaches	6

Aldrich & Chauncey (1990)
n = 130
Diagnostic Criteria:
Gender: [1]30/[2]35
Age:
Race:

Population Setting: community
Nationality: US
Other Sample Characteristics:
Method of Reporting: postal survey
Timeframe: current

Symptom	%
morning headaches[1]	7
morning headaches[2]	6

Lavie (1983)
n = 1,491
Diagnostic Criteria:
Gender:
Age: 41.9(11.5)
Race:

Population Setting: community
Nationality: Israel
Other Sample Characteristics:
Method of Reporting: self-report
Timeframe:

Symptom	%
ear and throat findings	26.8
excessive motility in sleep	40.3
frequent headaches	25.4

Symptom	%
heavy snoring	40.3
hypertension	7.4

Forero. Bauman, Young, et al. (1996)
n = 3,751
Diagnostic Criteria:
Gender:
Age: 41.9(11.5)
Race:

Population Setting: school
Nationality: Australia
Other Sample Characteristics:
Method of Reporting: self-report
Timeframe: current

Symptom	%
backaches weekly or more often	18.0
feeling dizzy weekly or more often	20.2

Symptom	%
feeling irritable (bad temper) weekly or more often	
feeling low/ depressed	30.4

feeling nervous weekly or more often	35.0
headaches weekly or more often	39.4

sleeping difficulties weekly or more often	34.0

Peckham & Butler (1978)
n = 11,845
Diagnostic Criteria:
Gender: 5,953/5,892
Age: 11
Race:

Population Setting: community
Nationality: UK
Other Sample Characteristics:
Method of Reporting: parent report
Timeframe: 1 year

Symptom	%
abdominal pain	10.7
headaches or migraine	15.1

Symptom	%
throat and/or ear infections	10.4
vomiting or bilious attacks	4.3

House, Dennis, Mogridge, et al.
(1991)
n = 111
Diagnostic Criteria:
Gender: 45/66
Age: 69.6(11.4); 30-86

Race:
Population Setting: community
Nationality: UK
Other Sample Characteristics:
Method of Reporting: self- report
Timeframe: 1 week

Symptom	%
body image	20
crying	27
fatigability	67
guilt	9
indecisiveness	25
irritability	38
lack of satisfaction	38
loss of appetite	16
loss of libido	35
pessimism	12
sadness	17

Symptom	%
self-accusation	27
self-hate	19
sense of failure	12
sense of punishment	7
sleep disturbance	50
social withdrawal	16
somatic preoccupation	17
suicidal ideas	2
weight loss	8
work inhibition	53

Roberts, Ingram, Lamar, et al. (1996)
n = 11
Diagnostic Criteria:
Gender:

Age: 70.8(8.8)
Race:
Population Setting: community
Nationality: US

Other Sample Characteristics:
Method of Reporting: cognitive
testing

Timeframe: current

Symptom	%
impaired comprehension of prosody	18
impaired elicitation of prosody	18

Symptom	%
impaired repetition of prosody	2

Hallman (1986)
n = 1,541
Diagnostic Criteria:
Gender: 0/1541
Age: 18-47
Race:

Population Setting: community
Nationality: Sweden
Other Sample Characteristics:
Method of Reporting: self-report
Timeframe: current

Symptom	%
abdomen swelling	62.2
anxiety	23.0
breast swelling	51.3

Symptom	%
depression	30.9
finger/leg swelling	19.7
irritability	62.7

Kashani, Rosenberg, & Reid (1989)
n = 70
Diagnostic Criteria:
Gender:
Age: 8
Race:

Population Setting: public schools
Nationality: US
Other Sample Characteristics:
Method of Reporting: [1]structured
interview; [2]self-report
Timeframe:

Symptom	%
agitation or hyperactivity when sad[1]	14.3
feeling very bored[2]	70.0
having horrible dreams[2]	54.3
having stomachaches[2]	81.4
irritable a lot[1]	18.6
more tired than before[1]	22.9
not having lots of energy[2]	37.1
not liking to go out and play[2]	17.1

Symptom	%
not looking forward to things as much as used to[2]	54.3
not sticking up for self[2]	45.7
thinking I won't get more of the good things out of life than others[2]	62.9
thinking there is no use trying to get what I want because I won't get it[2]	18.6
thinking tomorrow is unclear and confusing[2]	15.7

Kashani, Rosenberg, & Reid (1989)
n = 70
Diagnostic Criteria:
Gender:
Age: 12
Race:

Population Setting: public schools
Nationality: US
Other Sample Characteristics:
Method of Reporting: [1]structured
interview; [2]self-report
Timeframe:

Symptom	%
agitation or hyperactivity when sad[1]	21.4
doesn't care whether hurts self[1]	15.7
feeling very bored[2]	92.9
having horrible dreams[2]	27.1
having stomacheaches[2]	55.7
irritable a lot[1]	21.4
more tired than before[1]	15.7
not having lots of energy[2]	41.4
not liking to go out and play[2]	24.3

Symptom	%
not looking forward to things as much as used to[2]	47.1
not sticking up for self[2]	20
thinking I won't get more of the good things out of life than others[2]	54.3
thinking there is no use trying to get what I want because I won't get it[2]	10.0
thinking tomorrow is unclear and confusing[2]	12.9

Kashani, Rosenberg, & Reid (1989)
n = 70
Diagnostic Criteria:
Gender:
Age: 17
Race:

Population Setting: public schools
Nationality: US
Other Sample Characteristics:
Method of Reporting: [1]structured
interview; [2]self-report
Timeframe:

Symptom	%
agitation or hyperactivity when sad[1]	34.3
doesn't care whether hurts self[1]	37.1
feeling very bored[2]	84.3
having horrible dreams[2]	24.3
having stomachaches[2]	41.4
irritable a lot[1]	42.9
more tired than before[1]	34.3

Symptom	%
not having lots of energy[2]	67.1
not liking to go out and play[2]	48.6
not looking forward to things as much as used to[2]	31.4
not sticking up for self[2]	25.7
thinking I won't get more of the good things out of life than others[2]	34.3
thinking there is no use	2.9

trying to get what I want because I won't get it[2]	

thinking tomorrow is unclear and confusing[2]	34.3

Becker, Boller, Lopez, et al. (1994)
n = 101
Diagnostic Criteria:
Gender: 44/57
Age: 63.8(8.3); 46.2-81.9
Race:
Population Setting: behavioral neurology research clinic

Nationality:
Other Sample Characteristics:
Method of Reporting: [1]neurological exam; [2]semi structured psychiatric interview
Timeframe: current

Symptom	%
abnormal extraocular movements[1]	0
aggressiveness[2]	0
agitation[2]	14
agraphesthesia[1]	3
anxiety[2]	26
appetite decrease[2]	15
appetite increase[2]	7
auditory hallucinations[2]	0
bizarre behavior[2]	0
buccolingual praxis impaired[1]	3
cerebellar functions impaired[1]	0
cogwheeling[1]	0
decreased strength[1]	0
deep tendon reflexes abnormal[1]	2
delusions[2]	0
depressed mood[2]	11
dressing apraxia[1]	0
falling[1]	0
gait impaired[1]	2
gegenhalten[1]	3
general anxiety[2]	0
glabellar response[1]	0
grasp reflex[1]	0

Symptom	%
hypersomnia[2]	2
hyposomnia[2]	41
impaired olfaction[1]	2
incontinence[1]	0
irritability[2]	0
lack of energy[2]	29
lead pipe rigidity[1]	0
limb praxis impaired[1]	7
loss of interest[2]	10
loss of motivation[2]	6
motor impersistence[1]	0
myoclonus[1]	0
other cranial nerve abnormalities[1]	0
palmomental reflex[1]	7
panic attacks[2]	0
plantar response[1]	0
poor self-esteem[2]	2
rooting reflex[1]	0
sadness[2]	18
self-neglect[2]	0
situational anxiety[2]	2
snout reflex[1]	4
social withdrawal[2]	1
somatization[2]	0
stereoagnosis abnormal[1]	0

suicide[2]	1
sundowning[2]	0
suspiciousness[2]	0
syndromal major depression[2]	0
tremor[1]	1

unawareness of memory deficit[1]	1
visual and auditory hallucinations[2]	0
visual hallucinations[2]	0
wandering[2]	0

Hart, Bax, & Jenkins (1983)
n = 870
Diagnostic Criteria:
Gender:
Age: [1]1 year; [2]18 months; [3]2 years; [4]3 years; [5]4 1/2 years

Race:
Population Setting: community
Nationality: UK
Other Sample Characteristics:
Method of Reporting: parent report
Timeframe: 3 months

Symptom	%
night waking[1]	21
night waking[2]	17
night waking[3]	15
night waking[4]	12
night waking[5]	10
poor appetite[3]	11

Symptom	%
poor appetite[4]	16
poor appetite[5]	9
temper tantrums[3]	19
temper tantrums[4]	18
temper tantrums[5]	11

Breslau (1992)
n = 788
Diagnostic Criteria:
Gender:
Age: 21-30
Race:

Population Setting: community
Nationality:
Other Sample Characteristics:
Method of Reporting: structured interview
Timeframe: lifetime

Symptom	%
suicide attempt	2.2
thought a lot about death	26.2
thought about committing suicide	12.8

Symptom	%
wanted to die	3.8

Escobar, Burnam, Karno, et al. (1987)
n = 2,551
Diagnostic Criteria:

Gender:
Age:
Race: 1309/0/1,242/0/0/0
Population Setting: community

Nationality: US
Other Sample Characteristics:

Method of Reporting: structured
interview
Timeframe: lifetime

Symptom	%
abdominal pain	5.1
chest pain	4.7
dizziness	3.8
excessive gas	5.1

Symptom	%
fainting	4.5
painful periods	10.3
palpitations	5.9

Talley, Fett, Zinsmeister, et al. (1994)
n = 859
Diagnostic Criteria:
Gender: 405/454
Age: 30-49
Race: 859/0/0/0/0/0

Population Setting: community
Nationality: US
Other Sample Characteristics:
Method of Reporting: self-report
Timeframe: 1 year

Symptom	%
dyspepsia-Rome criteria	23.4
early satiety	0.4
frequent upper abdominal pain of moderate severity or more	12.0
frequent upper abdominal pain-any	16.3
gastric fullness postprandially often	1.7
heartburn once a week or more	11.6

Symptom	%
nausea once a month or more	9.3
retching once a month or more	0.4
upper abdominal bloating often without visible detention	0.6
upper abdominal discomfort often	4.1
vomiting once a month or more	0.6

Talley, Fett, Zinsmeister, et al. (1994)
n = 859
Diagnostic Criteria:
Gender: [1]405/[2]454
Age: 30-49
Race: 8594/0/0/0/0/0

Population Setting: community
Nationality: US
Other Sample Characteristics:
Method of Reporting: self-report
Timeframe: 1 year

Symptom	%
dyspepsia-Rome criteria[2]	26.1
dyspepsia-Rome criteria[1]	20.8

Symptom	%
early satiety often[1]	0.5
early satiety often[2]	0.3

frequent upper abdominal pain of moderate severity or more[1]	12.3
frequent upper abdominal pain of moderate severity or more[2]	11.8
frequent upper abdominal pain-any[1]	17.1
frequent upper abdominal pain-any[2]	15.6
gastric fullness postprandially often[1]	1.8
gastric fullness postprandially often[2]	1.7
heartburn once a week or more[1]	13.0
heartburn once a week or more[2]	10.3
nausea once a month or more[1]	8.9

nausea once a month or more[2]	9.8
retching once a month or more[1]	0.5
retching once a month or more[2]	0.3
upper abdominal bloating often without visible detention[1]	0.5
upper abdominal bloating often without visible detention[2]	0.6
upper abdominal discomfort often[1]	4.0
upper abdominal discomfort-often[2]	4.1
vomiting once a month or more[1]	0.7
vomiting once a month or more[2]	0.5

Fuhrer & Wessely (1995)
n = 3,784
Diagnostic Criteria:
Gender: 1,460/2,324
Age: 18-64
Race:

Population Setting: general practice patients
Nationality: France
Other Sample Characteristics:
Method of Reporting: [1]presenting complaint; [2]self-report
Timeframe: [1]current; [2]1 week

Symptom	%
fatigue[1]	7.6
lack of energy[2]	30.5

Symptom	%
lack of energy[2]	23.2
lack of energy[2]	35.1

Fuhrer & Wessely (1995)
n = 3,784
Diagnostic Criteria:
Gender: [1]1460/[2]2324
Age: 18-64
Race:

Population Setting: general practice patients
Nationality: France
Other Sample Characteristics:
Method of Reporting: presenting complaint
Timeframe: current

Symptom	%

fatigue[1]	6.8
fatigue[2]	8.1

Dick, Bland, & Newman (1994)
n = 3,211
Diagnostic Criteria:
Gender:
Age: 18+
Race:

Population Setting: community
Nationality: Canada
Other Sample Characteristics:
Method of Reporting: self-report
Timeframe: lifetime

Symptom	%
choking or smothering	1.6
dizzy or lightheaded	1.8
fear of dying, acting crazy	2.7
feeling faint	1.7
feelings of unreality	2.2
fingers or feet tingling	0.9

Symptom	%
heart pounding	4.7
hot or cold flushes	2.4
short of breath	2.5
sweating	4.0
tightness or pain in chest	2.0
trembling and shaking	3.7

Huerta-Franco & Malacaro (1993)
n = 502
Diagnostic Criteria:
Gender:
Age: 23.9
Race:

Population Setting: community
Nationality: Mexico
Other Sample Characteristics:
Method of Reporting: self-report
Timeframe: current

Symptom	%
abdominal bloating	30.9
anxiety	15.5
backache	28.3
breast tenderness	11.6
constipation	24.5
crying easily	16.1
depression	21.9
desire to be alone	13.0
desire to stay at home	21.3
dizziness	12.7
fatigue	35.8
headache	27.9

Symptom	%
inability to concentrate	17.7
increased appetite	19.7
insecurity	11.2
irritability	15.9
leg cramps	14.1
low abdominal pain	20.1
polydipsia	16.3
restlessness	10.6
sadness	26.5
tension	13.4
weakness	11.2

Waite, Broe, Creasey, et al. (1997)
n = 537
Diagnostic Criteria:
Gender: [1]282/[2]255
Age: 75-97
Race:

Population Setting: community
Nationality: Australia
Other Sample Characteristics:
Method of Reporting: physical exam
Timeframe: current

Symptom	%
cognitive impairment[1]	36
cognitive impairment[2]	39
gait ataxia[1]	42
gait ataxia[2]	57

Symptom	%
gait slowing[1]	18
gait slowing[2]	20
visual impairment[1]	45
visual impairment[2]	40

Wicki, Angst, & Merikangas (1992)
n = 457
Diagnostic Criteria:
Gender:
Age: 28
Race:

Population Setting: community
Nationality: Switzerland
Other Sample Characteristics:
Method of Reporting: semi-structured
interview
Timeframe: 1 year

Symptom	%
anxiety	28
appetite problems	34
back pain	54
cardiac complaints	23
circulatory complaints	23
depression	50
headache	59
hypochondriasis	21
hypomania	26
insomnia	47

Symptom	%
intestinal complaints	33
menstruation complaints	20
neurasthenia	25
obsessive-compulsive symptoms	8
panic	7
phobia	34
respiratory complaints	13
stomach complaints	37
suicide ideation or attempts	15

Klink, Dodge, & Quan (1994)
n = 1,358
Diagnostic Criteria:
Gender:
Age: 18+
Race: 1,358/0/0/0/0/0

Population Setting: community
Nationality: US
Other Sample Characteristics:
Method of Reporting: telephone
survey
Timeframe: current

Symptom	%
difficulty initiating or maintaining sleep	28.0
excessive daytime sleepiness	9.4

Hochstrasser & Angst (1996)
n = 91
Diagnostic Criteria:
Gender: [1]33/[2]58
Age: 20-21
Race:

Population Setting: community
Nationality: Switzerland
Other Sample Characteristics:
Method of Reporting: semi-structured interview
Timeframe: 1 year

Symptom	%
abdominal cramps[1]	72.7
abdominal cramps[2]	52.9
abdominal pain[1]	63.6
abdominal pain[2]	58.8
belching[1]	72.7
belching[2]	81.0
bloating[1]	63.6
bloating[2]	50.0
diarrhea[1]	36.4
diarrhea[2]	64.7
feeling of fullness[1]	81.8
feeling of fullness[2]	72.4
feelings of pressure/fullness[1]	63.6

Symptom	%
feelings of pressure/fullness[2]	50.0
nausea[1]	66.7
nausea[2]	48.3
obstipation[1]	54.6
obstipation[2]	29.4
stomach burning[1]	57.6
stomach burning[2]	70.7
stomach pain[1]	30.3
stomach pain[2]	36.2
stomach pressure[1]	66.7
stomach pressure[2]	63.8
vomiting[1]	84.8
vomiting[2]	81.0

Hochstrasser & Angst (1996)
n = 67
Diagnostic Criteria:
Gender: [1]17/[2]50
Age: 29-30
Race:

Population Setting: community
Nationality: Switzerland
Other Sample Characteristics:
Method of Reporting: semi-structured interview
Timeframe: 1 year

Symptom	%
abdominal pain[1]	45.5
abdominal pain[2]	48.9

Symptom	%
belching[1]	35.6
belching[2]	38.0

bloating[1]	63.6
bloating[2]	63.8
diarrhea[1]	54.6
diarrhea[2]	44.7
feelings of pressure/fullness[1]	54.6
feelings of pressure/fullness[2]	68.1
nausea[1]	41.2
nausea[2]	64.0

obstipation[1]	45.5
obstipation[2]	63.8
stomach burning[1]	52.9
stomach burning[2]	48.0
stomach pain[1]	47.1
stomach pain[2]	58.0
stomach pressure[1]	41.2
stomach pressure[2]	46.0
vomiting[1]	23.5
vomiting[2]	24.0

Schoenbach, Kaplan, Wagner, et al. (1983)
n = 504
Diagnostic Criteria:
Gender: [1]153/0; [2]104/0; [3]0/155; [4]0/92
Age: 12-16
Race: 0/92/0/0/0/0

Population Setting: public junior high school students
Nationality: US
Other Sample Characteristics:
Method of Reporting: self-report
Timeframe: 1 week

Symptom	%
bothered by things[1]	44
bothered by things[2]	61
bothered by things[3]	63
bothered by things[4]	69
could not get going[1]	45
could not get going[2]	59
could not get going[3]	56
could not get going[4]	49
could not shake blues[2]	56
could not shake blues[3]	56
could not shake blues[4]	56
could. not shake blues[1]	36
did not enjoy life[1]	53
did not enjoy life[2]	75
did not enjoy life[3]	58
did not enjoy life[4]	64
everything was an effort[1]	76
everything was an effort[2]	80
everything was an effort[3]	72

Symptom	%
everything was an effort[4]	72
felt depressed[1]	45
felt depressed[2]	58
felt depressed[3]	59
felt depressed[4]	63
felt fearful[1]	34
felt fearful[2]	52
felt fearful[3]	44
felt fearful[4]	64
felt lonely[1]	38
felt lonely[2]	66
felt lonely[3]	47
felt lonely[4]	46
felt people disliked me[1]	39
felt people disliked me[2]	55
felt people disliked me[3]	52
felt people disliked me[4]	43
felt sad[1]	39
felt sad[2]	59

Symptom	%
felt sad[3]	51
felt sad[4]	42
had crying spells[1]	18
had crying spells[2]	41
had crying spells[3]	37
had crying spells[4]	35
life had been a failure[1]	19
life had been a failure[2]	51
life had been a failure[3]	34
life had been a failure[4]	46
not feel like eating[1]	30
not feel like eating[2]	55
not feel like eating[3]	46
not feel like eating[4]	51
not happy[1]	60
not happy[2]	79
not happy[3]	57
not happy[4]	73
not hopeful about future[4]	74
not hopeful about the future[1]	68
not hopeful about the future[2]	85
not hopeful about the future[3]	76

Symptom	%
not just as good as others[1]	68
not just as good as others[2]	71
not just as good as others[3]	75
not just as good as others[4]	68
people were unfriendly[1]	49
people were unfriendly[2]	51
people were unfriendly[3]	48
people were unfriendly[4]	46
sleep was restless[1]	37
sleep was restless[2]	52
sleep was restless[3]	46
sleep was restless[4]	63
talked less than usual[1]	50
talked less than usual[2]	78
talked less than usual[3]	57
talked less than usual[4]	69
trouble keeping mind on things[1]	62
trouble keeping mind on things[2]	71
trouble keeping mind on things[3]	78
trouble keeping mind on things[4]	64

FAMILY PRACTICE

Fox, Lees-Haley, Earnest, et al. (1995)
n = 124
Diagnostic Criteria:
Gender: 44/80
Age: 48

Race:
Population Setting: HMO patients
Nationality: US
Other Sample Characteristics:
Method of Reporting: self-report
Timeframe: 2 years

Symptom	%
concentration	40
concentration	40
dizziness	27
ear ringing	20

Symptom	%
fatigue	59
fatigue	59
headache	50
impatience	35

impatience	35
irritability	44
irritability	44
memory	33

noise sensitivity	15
noise sensitivity	15
visual	26
visual	26

Amodei, Elkin, Burge, et al. (1994)
n = 60
Diagnostic Criteria:
Gender: 30/30
Age: 40.5 (13.0)
Race: 3/3/54/0/0

Population Setting: family practice
clinic
Nationality: US
Other Sample Characteristics:
Method of Reporting: structured
clinical interview
Timeframe: [1]30 days, [2]lifetime

Symptom	%
anxiety[1]	16.7
anxiety[2]	28.3
depression[1]	13.3
depression[2]	30.0
hallucinations[1]	0.0
hallucinations[2]	5.0
prescribed medications[1]	5.0
prescribed medications[2]	21.7

Symptom	%
suicidal thoughts[1]	3.3
suicidal thoughts[2]	13.3
suicide attempts[1]	0.0
suicide attempts[2]	8.3
trouble concentrating[1]	11.7
trouble concentrating[2]	16.7
violent behavior[1]	3.3
violent behavior[2]	10.0

GENERAL PRACTICE

Doull, Williams, Freezer, et al.
(1996)
n = 4,830
Diagnostic Criteria:
Gender: 2,508/2,293
Age: 8.04 (.86)

Race:
Population Setting: general medical
patients
Nationality: UK
Other Sample Characteristics:
Method of Reporting: parent report
Timeframe: 12 months

Symptom	%
chronic cough	10
chronic cough and wheeze	7.6

Symptom	%
wheezing	5.5

Tse, Cooper, Bridges-Webb, et al.
(1993)
n = 1,933
Diagnostic Criteria:
Gender:
Age: 8.04
Race:

Population Setting: general medicine
outpatients
Nationality: Australia
Other Sample Characteristics:
Method of Reporting: self report
Timeframe: [1]1 year, [2]lifetime

Symptom	%
wheeze[1]	19

Symptom	%
wheeze[2]	23

INTERNAL MEDICINE

Fox, Lees-Haley, Earnest, et al.
(1995)
n = 190
Diagnostic Criteria:
Gender: 57/133
Age: 49.4

Race: 268/88/66/7/0/9
Population Setting: HMO patients
Nationality: US
Other Sample Characteristics:
Method of Reporting: self-report
Timeframe: 2 years

Symptoms	%
concentration	17
dizziness	24
ear ringing	21
fatigue	33
headache	38

Symptoms	%
impatience	26
irritability	27
memory	23
noise sensitivity	13
visual	27

LITIGANTS

Lees-Haley & Brown (1993)
n = 170
Diagnostic Criteria:
Gender: 90/80
Age: 39 (11.1)
Race:
Population Setting: litigation
claimants

Nationality: US
Other Sample Characteristics:
emotional distress or industrial stress
claims, non-neurological injuries,
litigants
Method of Reporting: self-report
Timeframe: since injury

Symptoms	%
anxiety or nervousness	93

Symptoms	%
back pain	80

bleeding	11
broken bone or bones	2
bumping into things	21
concentration problems	78
confusion	59
constipation	29
depression	89
diarrhea	2
dizziness	44
elbow pain	21
fatigue (mental or physical)	79
feeling disorganized	61
foot pain	24
headaches	88
hearing problems	29
impatience	65
impotence	15
irritability	77
loss of efficiency in carrying out everyday tasks	56

loss of interest	60
memory problems	53
nausea	38
neck pain	74
numbness	39
restlessness	62
seizures	4
sexual problems	41
shoulder pain	55
sleeping problems	92
speech problems	18
trembling or tremors	30
trouble reading	24
visual problems, blurring, or seeing double	32
word finding problems, not finding the word you want, using the wrong word	34
worried about health	77

MEDICAL AND DENTAL STUDENTS

Blau (1990)
n = 327
Diagnostic Criteria:
Gender: 198/129
Age: 18-32
Race:

Population Setting: medical and dental school
Nationality: US
Other Sample Characteristics:
Method of Reporting: self-report
Timeframe: lifetime

Symptom	%
has headaches	97.9
headache due to alcohol	38.5
headache due to excessive cold	2.1
headache due to excessive heat	36.7

Symptoms	%
headache due to excessive light	27.2
headache due to excessive noise	29.2
headache due to excessive sleep	23.5

headache due to exercise	8.3
headache due to hunger	14.1
headache due to ice-cream	10.7
headache due to insufficient sleep	38.8
headache due to menstruation	19.4
headache due to mental stress	38.8

headache due to other causes	19.0
headache due to reading	31.5
headache due to shopping	12.8
headache due to travel	19.6
headache due to watching a movie	5.2

NEUROLOGY

Fox, Lees-Haley, Earnest, et al.
(1995)
n = 104
Diagnostic Criteria:
Gender: 60/44
Age: 50.4

Race:
Population Setting: HMO patients
Nationality: US
Other Sample Characteristics:
Method of Reporting: self-report
Timeframe: 2 years

Symptom	%
concentration	34
dizziness	30
ear ringing	22
fatigue	52
headache	49

Symptoms	%
impatience	38
irritability	41
memory	36
noise sensitivity	16
visual	29

NONSMOKERS

Tashkin, Coulson, Clark, et al. (1987)
n = 97
Diagnostic Criteria:
Gender: [1]59/[2]38
Age: [1]31.9; [2]32
Race:

Population Setting: community
Nationality: US
Other Sample Characteristics:
Method of Reporting: structured
telephone interview
Timeframe: 1 year

Symptom	%
acute bronchitic episode lasting > 3 weeks[1]	18.0

Symptom	%
acute bronchitic episode lasting > 3 weeks[2]	2.9

cough present on most days[1]	0.0
cough present on most days[2]	2.9
shortness of breath[1]	0.0
shortness of breath[2]	5.7

sputum present on most days[1]	0.0
sputum present on most days[2]	14.3
wheeze present >21 days[1]	3.6
wheeze present >21 days[2]	14.3

NORMAL

Chee & Sachder (1997)
$\underline{n} = 45$
Diagnostic Criteria:
Gender: 22/23
Age: 20.7 (5.3)
Race:

Population Setting: health service workers
Nationality: Australia
Other Sample Characteristics:
Method of Reporting: interviewer rating
Timeframe: [1]lifetime; [2]during tics

Symptom	%
eye tics[1]	0.0
face/head tics[1]	2.2
itch/tickle/insect crawling sensations[2]	2.2
lower limb tics[1]	4.4
neck tics[1]	0.0

Symptom	%
sensory tics[1]	8.9
tightness/tension[2]	0.0
tingling/crinking/ electrical sensations[2]	0.0
torso tics[1]	0.0
upper limb tics[1]	2.2

Merello, Sabe, Teson, et al. (1994)
$\underline{n} = 20$
Diagnostic Criteria:
Gender: 7/13
Age: 70.9 (8.1)
Race:

Population Setting: community
Nationality: Argentina
Other Sample Characteristics:
Method of Reporting: neurological exam
Timeframe: current

Symptom	%
abnormal gait	10
abnormal posture	25
abnormal speech	0
action tremor	5
altering movements	5
body bradykinesia	5
finger tapping	10

Symptom	%
hand movements	5
leg agility	5
masked face	25
postural instability	5
resting tremor	0
rigidity	40
rising from a chair	5

Moorey & Soni (1994)
n = 30
Diagnostic Criteria:
Gender: 14/16
Age: 41; 18-62
Race:

Population Setting: community
Nationality: UK
Other Sample Characteristics:
Method of Reporting:
Timeframe:

Symptom	%
anxiety	7

Weiss, Hechtman, Milroy, et al.
(1985)
n = 42
Diagnostic Criteria:
Gender: 38/4
Age: 25.1; 21-32

Race:
Population Setting: community
Nationality: Canada
Other Sample Characteristics:
Method of Reporting:
Timeframe: 3 years

Symptom	%
interpersonal problems	75.0
neurotic problems	79.0
psychotic problems	8.2
sexual problems	20.0

Symptom	%
suicidal attempts	0.0
suicidal thoughts	26.8
symptoms related to	68.2

DeSmet, Ruberg, Sedaru,et al. (1982)
n = 41
Diagnostic Criteria:
Gender:
Age: 60.7 (1.3)
Race:
Population Setting: neurology and
neuropsychology clinic inpatients

Nationality: France
Other Sample Characteristics: taking
anticholinergic drugs
Method of Reporting: neurological
exam
Timeframe: current

Symptom	%
confusional state	9.8

Ackerman, Dykman, & Peters (1977)
n = 31
Diagnostic Criteria:
Gender:
Age: 14

Race:
Population Setting:
Nationality: US
Other Sample Characteristics: follow-
up

Method of Reporting: rater report   Timeframe: current

Symptom	%
excessively fidgety	6.5
extremely slow moving	0.0
intermittently fidgety	0.0

Symptom	%
overtalkative	3.2
sullen	6.5

Mavrikakis, Sfikakis, Kontoyannis, et al. (1991)
n = 350
Diagnostic Criteria:
Gender: 141/209
Age: 65.7; 34-87

Race:
Population Setting: inpatients
Nationality: Greece
Other Sample Characteristics:
Method of Reporting: X-ray
Timeframe: current

Symptom	%
calcific shoulder periarthritis	10

Muller, Montoya, Shandry, et al. (1994)
n = 45
Diagnostic Criteria:
Gender: 20/25
Age: 44.7 (15.4); 24-81
Race:

Population Setting: community
Nationality: Germany
Other Sample Characteristics: [1]"day 2"; [2]"day 30"
Method of Reporting: self-report
Timeframe: current

Symptom	%
chest tightness[1]	20
chest tightness[2]	10
clammy hands/feet[1]	5
clammy hands/feet[2]	5
cold hands/feet[1]	25
cold hands/feet[2]	10
dizziness[1]	15
dizziness[2]	15
headache[1]	25
headache[2]	20
nausea[1]	10
nausea[2]	5
pounding heart[1]	35

Symptom	%
pounding heart[2]	15
restlessness[1]	30
restlessness[2]	30
shortness of breath[1]	15
shortness of breath[2]	15
sleep disturbance[1]	20
sleep disturbance[2]	20
throbbing temples[1]	15
throbbing temples[2]	10
tiredness[1]	60
tiredness[2]	50
warmth[1]	10
warmth[2]	15

Hendren, Hodde-Vargas, Yeo, et al.
(1995)
n = 13
Diagnostic Criteria:
Gender: 7/6
Age: 29.7(19.4)
Race:

Population Setting: public school
students or pediatric outpatients
Nationality:
Other Sample Characteristics:
Method of Reporting:
neuropsychological tests
Timeframe:

Symptom	%
impaired frontal ability	40
impaired nonverbal ability	0

Symptom	%
impaired verbal ability	0
impaired verbal memory	10

Noyes, Cook, & Garvey (1990)
n = 30
Diagnostic Criteria:
Gender: 12/18
Age:
Race:

Population Setting: drug study
subjects
Nationality: US
Other Sample Characteristics:
Method of Reporting: self-report
Timeframe: 1 week

Symptom	%
belching	40.0
bloating	3.3
constipation	6.7
diarrhea	6.7
dry mouth	6.7
heartburn	10.0
lower abdominal pain	6.7
lump in throat	6.7

Symptom	%
nausea	6.7
passing of gas	46.7
poor appetite	0.0
trouble eating	0.0
trouble swallowing	3.3
upper abdominal pain	3.3
vomiting	0.0

Lydiard, Greenwald, Weissman, et al.
(1994)
n = 8973
Diagnostic Criteria:
Gender:
Age: 18+
Race:

Population Setting: community
Nationality: US
Other Sample Characteristics:
Method of Reporting: structured
interview
Timeframe: lifetime

Symptom	%
abdominal pain	4.7

Symptom	%
constipation	7.5

diarrhea	2.9
frequent vomiting	1.5
nausea without vomiting	3.2

sickness from certain foods	2.4
stomach bloating	6.6
symptoms of IBS	0.7

Fox, Lees-Haley, Earnest, et al.
(1995)
n = 292
Diagnostic Criteria:
Gender: 148/144
Age: 34.7

Race:
Population Setting: HMO patients
Nationality: US
Other Sample Characteristics:
Method of Reporting: self-report
Timeframe: 2 years

Symptom	%
concentration	19
dizziness	24
ear ringing	18
fatigue	34
headache	43

Symptom	%
impatience	24
irritability	33
memory	18
noise sensitivity	11
visual	24

Glosser, Wolfe, Kliner-Krenzel, et al.
(1994)
n = 31
Diagnostic Criteria:
Gender: 17/14
Age: 71.2 (10.0)
Race:

Population Setting: neurology clinic
outpatients
Nationality: US
Other Sample Characteristics:
Method of Reporting: structured
interview
Timeframe: current

Symptoms	%
anxiety	0
cooperation	0
depression	0

Symptoms	%
motor slowing	0
psychosis	0

Johnson, DeLuca & Natelson (1996)
n = 33
Diagnostic Criteria:
Gender: 2/31
Age: 34.5(1.7)
Race:

Population Setting: community
Nationality: US
Other Sample Characteristics:
Method of Reporting: structured
interview
Timeframe: lifetime

Symptom	%
6 months of pain	0
abdominal pain	3
back pain	0
blurred vision	0
chest pain	0
constipation	3
crying spells	18
diarrhea	0
dizziness	3
double vision	9
excess gas	6
excessive menstruation	3
extremity pain	5
fainting	9
food intolerance	3
headaches	16
hopelessness	9

Symptom	%
irregular menstruation	9
joint pain	3
loss of feeling	0
lump in throat	3
menstrual pain	6
missed menstruation	6
muscle weakness	0
nausea	0
painful intercourse	0
sexual difficulties	3
sexual indifference	34
shortness of breath	0
sickliness throughout life	0
sudden weight change	0
tachycardia	25
time off due to illness	0
trouble walking	0

Krupp, Jandorf, Coyle, et al. (1993)
n = 40
Diagnostic Criteria:
Gender: 12/28
Age: 32(10)
Race:

Population Setting: community
Nationality:
Other Sample Characteristics:
Method of Reporting: self-report
Timeframe: previous night

Symptom	%
bothered by early morning waking	0
slept badly	5

Symptom	%
slept lightly	10
still felt drowsy upon awakening	35

Flament, Koby, Rapoport, et al. (1990)
n = 40
Diagnostic Criteria:
Gender: 12/28
Age: 18.5(2.1); 14-22
Race:

Population Setting: community
Nationality: US
Other Sample Characteristics:
Method of Reporting: structured interview
Timeframe: lifetime

Symptom	%
suicide attempts	4

Watkins, Williamson, & Falkowski
(1989)
n = 30
Diagnostic Criteria:
Gender: 0/30
Age: 33.5; 25-42
Race:

Population Setting: college
undergraduates
Nationality: US
Other Sample Characteristics:
Method of Reporting: self-report
Timeframe: 2 months

Symptom	%
appetite	0.0
autonomic reactions	0.0
behavior change	6.7
concentration	0.0

Symptom	%
negative affect	6.7
pain	0.0
water retention	36.7

Gerbaldo & Thaker (1991)
n = 17
Diagnostic Criteria:
Gender: 9/8
Age: 34(10)
Race:

Population Setting:
Nationality:
Other Sample Characteristics:
Method of Reporting: experiment
Timeframe: current

Symptom	%
photophilic behavior	0

Weissman, Klerman, Markowitz, et
al. (1988)
n = 12,233
Diagnostic Criteria:
Gender: 4844/7389
Age: 18+
Race: 8245/263/0/0/0/1246

Population Setting: community
Nationality: US
Other Sample Characteristics:
Method of Reporting: structured
interview
Timeframe:

Symptom	%
felt like you want to die	3
suicide attempts	1

Symptom	%
thought about suicide	4

Heaton, Ghosh, & Braddon (1991)   n = 27

Diagnostic Criteria:
Gender: 0/27
Age: 29; 21-38
Race:
Population Setting: community

Nationality: UK
Other Sample Characteristics:
Method of Reporting: self-report
diary
Timeframe: 1 month

Symptom	%
abdominal pain	81
bloating	93
defecation urgent	11
excessively frequent defecation	7
incomplete evacuation of bowel movement	15

Symptom	%
infrequent defecation	19
irregularity	0
straining to finish	11
straining to start	63

Linet, Stewart, Celentano, et al.
(1989)
$\underline{n}$ = 3158
Diagnostic Criteria:
Gender: [1]1523/[2]1635
Age: 12-17
Race:
Population Setting: community

Nationality: US
Other Sample Characteristics:
subjects experienced at least one
headache in the 5 year period before
the interview
Method of Reporting: interview
Timeframe: 4 weeks

Symptom	%
migraine[1]	3.8
migraine[2]	6.6

Linet, Stewart, Celentano, et al.
(1989)
$\underline{n}$ = 3210
Diagnostic Criteria:
Gender: [1]1480/[2]1730
Age: 18-23
Race:
Population Setting: community

Nationality: US
Other Sample Characteristics:
subjects experienced at least one
headache in the 5 year period before
the interview
Method of Reporting: interview
Timeframe: 4 weeks

Symptom	%
migraine[1]	3.0
migraine[2]	6.7

Linet, Stewart, Celentano, et al.
(1989)
n = 3081
Diagnostic Criteria:
Gender: [1]1391/[2]1690
Age: 24-29
Race:
Population Setting: community

Nationality: US
Other Sample Characteristics:
subjects experienced at least one
headache in the 5 year period before
the interview
Method of Reporting: interview
Timeframe: 4 weeks

Symptom	%
migraine[1]	2.2
migraine[2]	8.8

Linet, Stewart, Celentano, et al.
(1989)
n = 2054
Diagnostic Criteria:
Gender: [1]851/[2]1203
Age: 12-17

Race:
Population Setting: community
Nationality: US
Other Sample Characteristics:
Method of Reporting: interview
Timeframe: 4 weeks

Symptom	%
awakened from sleep by headache[1]	5.4
awakened from sleep by headache[2]	5.5
feeling of a tight band around the head during headache[1]	17.1
feeling of a tight band around the head during headache[2]	14.1
headache occurred after sleeping longer than usual[1]	8.8
headache occurred after sleeping longer than usual[2]	8.4
nausea/ vomiting during headache[1]	8.2

Symptom	%
nausea/ vomiting during headache[2]	10.5
numbness/ tingling/ peculiar feeling in one arm/ leg during headache[1]	3.1
numbness/ tingling/ peculiar feeling in one arm/ leg during headache[2]	2.1
pain in back of head, neck or shoulders during headache[1]	15.2
pain in back of head, neck or shoulders during headache[2]	17.4
partial loss of vision before headache[1]	2.4
partial loss of vision before headache[2]	2.4
spots/ lines/ heat waves before headache[1]	8.3

spots/ lines/ heat waves before headache[2]	10.3
unilateral pain during headache[1]	8.2
unilateral pain during headache[2]	30.1
unilateral soreness of	2.6

scalp during headache[1]	
unilateral soreness of scalp during headache[2]	3.9

Linet, Stewart, Celentano, et al. (1989)
$\underline{n}$ = 2195
Diagnostic Criteria:
Gender: [1]840/[2]1355
Age: 18-23

Race:
Population Setting: community
Nationality: US
Other Sample Characteristics:
Method of Reporting: interview
Timeframe: 4 weeks

Symptom	%
awakened from sleep by headache[1]	3.9
awakened from sleep by headache[2]	4.5
feeling of a tight band around the head during headache[1]	15.3
feeling of a tight band around the head during headache[2]	14.1
headache occurred after sleeping longer than usual[1]	9.1
headache occurred after sleeping longer than usual[2]	10.4
nausea/ vomiting during headache[1]	6.1
nausea/ vomiting during headache[2]	13.5
numbness/ tingling/ peculiar feeling in one arm/ leg during headache[1]	2.4
numbness/ tingling/ peculiar feeling in one arm/ leg during headache[2]	2.4

Symptom	%
pain in back of head, neck or shoulders during headache[1]	18.6
pain in back of head, neck or shoulders during headache[2]	23.5
partial loss of vision before headache[1]	2.8
partial loss of vision before headache[2]	2.4
spots/ lines/ heat waves before headache[1]	6.2
spots/ lines/ heat waves before headache[2]	7.5
unilateral pain during headache[1]	23.5
unilateral pain during headache[2]	26.2
unilateral soreness of scalp during headache[1]	2.2
unilateral soreness of scalp during headache[2]	3.6

Linet, Stewart, Celentano, et al.
(1989)
n = 2126
Diagnostic Criteria:
Gender: [1]819/[2]1307
Age: 24-29

Race:
Population Setting: community
Nationality: US
Other Sample Characteristics:
Method of Reporting: interview
Timeframe: 4 weeks

Symptom	%
awakened from sleep by headache[1]	2.1
awakened from sleep by headache[2]	7.7
feeling of a tight band around the head during headache[1]	12.3
feeling of a tight band around the head during headache[2]	16.0
headache occurred after sleeping longer than usual[1]	9.1
headache occurred after sleeping longer than usual[2]	9.3
nausea/ vomiting during headache[1]	6.1
nausea/ vomiting during headache[2]	18.0
numbness/ tingling/ peculiar feeling in one arm/ leg during headache[1]	2.3
numbness/ tingling/ peculiar feeling in one arm/ leg during headache[2]	3.8

Symptom	%
pain in back of head, neck or shoulders during headache[1]	23.0
pain in back of head, neck or shoulders during headache[2]	27.0
partial loss of vision before headache[1]	1.9
partial loss of vision before headache[2]	1.5
spots/ lines/ heat waves before headache[1]	4.7
spots/ lines/ heat waves before headache[2]	8.6
unilateral pain during headache[1]	23.4
unilateral pain during headache[2]	27.0
unilateral soreness of scalp during headache[1]	3.0
unilateral soreness of scalp during headache[2]	6.7

Steinhausen, Nestler, & Spohr (1982)
n = 28
Diagnostic Criteria:
Gender: 16/12
Age: 39-133 months
Race:

Population Setting: pediatric clinics, foster homes, private pediatric practices
Nationality: West Germany
Other Sample Characteristics:
Method of Reporting: developmental history
Timeframe: lifetime

Symptom	%
behavior disorders during preschool period	30
failure to thrive	5
problems of suck	10
retarded motor development	18

Symptom	%
retarded speech development	22
retarded toilet training	36

Mannuzza,Gittleman,Bonagura, et al (1988)
n = 52
Diagnostic Criteria:
Gender:
Age: 18.4 (1.5); 16-23
Race:
Population Setting: medical center outpatients

Nationality: US
Other Sample Characteristics: diagnosed as hyperactive between 6-12 yrs. of age
Method of Reporting: structured interview
Timeframe: [1]during high school; [2]between ages 16-18; [3]after age 18

Symptom	%
"on the go" driven by a motor[2]	21
acts on things immediately[2]	17
actually hit someone when angry[2]	27
arrested[1]	25
arrested[1]	2
attentional difficulties[3]	20
breaking & entering[1]	12
chronic lateness[1]	12
destroyed property[1]	12
difficulty keeping mind on interesting materials[2]	12
difficulty sitting or with quiet activities[2]	15
driving problems (ex. accident) [1]	2
easily distracted at work/school[2]	17
expelled from school[1]	2

Symptom	%
fighting[1]	2
fired[1]	0
frequent arguing at home[1]	12
hyperactivity[3]	13
illegal income[3]	0
impulsivity[3]	17
job or school problems[1]	2
job problems[1]	19
makes decisions too quickly[2]	23
many decisions regretted[2]	15
mind frequently somewhere else[2]	23
moderate to extreme attentional difficulties[3]	20
no alcohol related problems[1]	96
no conduct problems[1]	58
no conduct problems[1]	73
no regular home for more than 1 month[3]	0

often called impatient by others[2]	21
often got into arguments[2]	46
others complain of his not paying attention[2]	13
others said he had a violent temper[2]	25
over $100[1]	6
overall severity[2]	52
persistent lying[3]	0
physical fighting[3]	3
pranks[1]	12
smashed or threw things[2]	23
sued for bad debts[3]	0
suspended or expelled[1]	21
temper caused trouble w/police or at school[2]	19

theft (excluding minor) [1]	21
threatened to hurt someone[2]	19
threw objects at cars/people[1]	8
trouble concentrating or paying attention[2]	21
trouble finishing things[2]	12
trouble for fighting[1]	4
truancy[1]	25
use of alias[3]	0
use of weapon[3]	0
vagrancy[3]	0
vandalism[1]	2
verbal abuse to teachers[1]	13
very restless & fidgety[2]	19
violation of rules[1]	19

Mannuzza,Gittleman,Bonagura, et al (1988)
n = 80
Diagnostic Criteria:
Gender:
Age: 19 (1.6); 16-23
Race:

Population Setting: medical center outpatients
Nationality: US
Other Sample Characteristics:
Method of Reporting: structured interview
Timeframe: [1]during high school; [2]between ages 16-18; [3]after age 18

Symptom	%
acts on things immediately[2]	19
actually hit someone when angry[2]	33
arrested[1]	23
arrested[2]	3
attentional difficulties[3]	5
breaking & entering[1]	10
chronic lateness[1]	18
destroyed property[1]	16
difficulty keeping his mind on interesting materials[2]	4

Symptom	%
difficulty sitting, or with quiet activities[2]	6
driving problems (ex. accident) [1]	6
easily distracted at work/school[2]	6
expelled from school[1]	3
fighting[1]	6
fired[1]	0
frequent arguing at home[1]	24
hyperactivity[3]	5
illegal income[3]	9
impulsivity[3]	12

job or school problems[1]	4
job problems[1]	8
makes decisions too quickly[2]	18
many decisions regretted[2]	19
mind frequently somewhere else[2]	8
moderate to extreme attentional difficulty[3]	5
no alcohol related problems[1]	89
no conduct problems[1]	63
no conduct problems[1]	68
no regular home for more than 1 month[3]	0
often called impatient by others[2]	13
often got into arguments[2]	60
others complain of his not paying attention[2]	5
others said he had a violent temper[2]	33
"On the go" driven by a motor[2]	9
over $100[1]	3
overall severity[2]	63

persistent lying[3]	3
physical fighting[3]	9
pranks[1]	5
smashed or threw things[2]	24
sued for bad debts[3]	0
suspended or expelled[1]	18
temper caused trouble with police or at school[2]	13
theft (excluding minor)[1]	21
threatened to hurt someone[2]	26
threw objects at cars/people[1]	10
trouble concentrating or paying attention[2]	8
trouble finishing things[2]	5
trouble for fighting[1]	8
truancy[1]	31
use of a weapon[3]	0
use of alias[3]	0
vagrancy[3]	0
vandalism[1]	1
verbal abuse to teachers[1]	9
very restless & fidgety[2]	10
violation of rules[1]	11

Wheatley, Balter, Levine, et al. (1975)
n = 174
Diagnostic Criteria:
Gender: 98/76
Age:
Race:

Population Setting: general medical outpatients
Nationality: UK
Other Sample Characteristics:
Method of Reporting: self-report
Timeframe: 12 months

Symptom	%
anger-hostility	21.5
anxiety	58.0

Symptom	%
depression	33.5

Krupp, Alvarez, LaRocca, et al. (1988)

n = 32
Diagnostic Criteria:

Gender: 11/21
Age: 39 (11)
Race:
Population Setting: MS patient
relatives and hospital workers

Nationality: US
Other Sample Characteristics:
Method of Reporting: self-report
Timeframe: current

Symptom	%
bothered by fatigue	51

Fava, Rosenbaum, McCarthy, et al.
(1991)
n = 29
Diagnostic Criteria:
Gender: 11/18
Age: 18-35
Race:

Population Setting: health workers
and students
Nationality: US
Other Sample Characteristics:
Method of Reporting: self-report
Timeframe:

Symptom	%
anger attacks	21

McCormick, Kukull, vanBelle, et al.
(1994)
n = 129
Diagnostic Criteria:
Gender: 48/81
Age: 77(6)
Race: 124/0/0/0/0/5

Population Setting: HMO patients
Nationality:
Other Sample Characteristics:
Method of Reporting: medical
records
Timeframe: 1st symptom

Symptom	%
agitation	1.6
confusion	0.8
cough	28.0
depression	11.0
forgetfulness	1.6
gastrointestinal symptoms	44.0
genitourinary symptoms	19.0
hard of hearing	16.0

Symptom	%
hypersomnia	0.0
joint pain	57.0
memory problems	0.8
rash	24.0
thinking problems	1.6
vision problems	24.0
weight loss	2.0

OCCUPATIONAL

Ng, Lim, & Win (1992)
n = 15
Diagnostic Criteria:
Gender: 15/0
Age: 34.2 (5.36) 26-41
Race: 0/0/0/15/0/0

Population Setting: non-solvent
exposed paint factory workers
Nationality: Singapore
Other Sample Characteristics:
Method of Reporting: structured
interview
Timeframe

Symptoms	%
abnormally tired	6.7
depressed	13.3
difficulty buttoning	6.7
difficulty in concentration	6.7
difficulty walking in dark	6.7
dry skin	6.7
feel afraid w/out real danger	6.7
feel sleepy during the day	20.0
get high at work	0.0
hard to get meaning from reading	6.7
headache at least once a week	0.0
insomnia	6.7
irritable	13.3
numbness of lower limbs	6.7
numbness of upper limbs	6.7

Symptoms	%
often have to go back and check things	6.7
often have to make notes to remember	13.3
painful tingling in extremities	13.3
palpitations w/out exertion	0.0
perspire w/out particular reason	13.3
poor appetite	0.0
short memory	13.3
skin rash	0.0
told to have short memory	6.7
vertigo	0.0
wake up at night	6.7
weakness of lower limbs	0.0
weakness of upper limbs	0.0

Orbaek, Risberg, Rosen, et al. (1985)
n = 50
Diagnostic Criteria:
Gender:
Age:
Race:

Population Setting: sugar refinery
workers
Nationality: Sweden
Other Sample Characteristics:
Method of Reporting: [1]neurological
exam; [2]self-report
Timeframe: current

Symptom	%
alcohol incontinence[2]	8
cardiac palpitations[2]	4
chest oppression[2]	4

Symptoms	%
clinical signs of slight neuropathy[1]	4
concentration difficulties[2]	6

creeping paresthesia[2]	2
depressive feelings[2]	0
dyspepsia[2]	26
excessive sweating[2]	4
fatigue[2]	2
headache[2]	8
irritability[2]	4
mental exhaustion during workday[2]	28
mood lability[2]	2
numbness[2]	0

physical exhaustion[2]	10
recent memory failure[2]	10
restless legs[2]	0
sexual dysfunction[2]	0
sleep disturbances[2]	6
tingling paresthesia[2]	4
tremor[2]	6
vertigo[2]	0

Lundberg, Michelsen, Nise, et al. (1995)
n = 71
Diagnostic Criteria:
Gender:
Age:
Race:

Population Setting: carpenters
Nationality: Sweden
Other Sample Characteristics:
Method of Reporting: [1]self-report, [2]MRI, EEG[3]
Timeframe: [1]during work; [2]current

Symptom	%
abdominal pain[1]	7.0
abnormal EEG (current)[3]	11.0
abnormal finger-nose[1]	35.2
abnormal knee-heel[1]	56.3
abnormal left vibration sensitivity (toe)[1]	1.4
abnormal line walking[1]	41.0
abnormal right vibration sensitivity (toe)[1]	2.8
abnormal romberg[1]	51.0
abnormal tremor[1]	7.0
acid eructation[1]	9.0
anger, hostility[1]	24.0
anxiety nervousness[1]	14.1
awake long before falling asleep on weekends[1]	65.0
awake long before falling asleep on weeknights[1]	55.0

Symptoms	%
can't stand smell of solvents[1]	21.1
confusion[1]	28.2
decreased speed[1]	17.0
depression-dejection[1]	24.0
disturbed, uneasy sleep[1]	115.0
easily tired[1]	46.5
emotional lability[1]	15.5
expansion of areas filled w/cerebrospinal fluid[2]	40.0
fatigue[1]	24.0
feeling tired when waking up[1]	92.0
focal morphological changes[2]	6.7
frequent headache[1]	14.1
heavy snoring[1]	48.0
impaired balance in darkness[1]	5.6

impaired balance in daylight[1]	10.0
impaired concentration[1]	10.0
impaired intellect[1]	0.0
impaired memory[1]	31.0
impaired sense of smell[1]	23.0
impaired sense of taste[1]	7.0
involuntary dozing during leisure time[1]	61.0
involuntary dozing during work[1]	43.7
irritability[1]	15.5
lightheadedness[1]	1.0
lightheadedness[1]	1.0
loss of initiative[1]	6.0
lower alcohol tolerance[1]	27.0
mood change[1]	7.0
recovery[1]	61.0

reduced vigor[1]	24.0
rotational vertigo[1]	15.5
sexual problems[1]	18.3
sleep apnea[1]	51.0
sleep quality[1]	57.7
sleeping problems[1]	8.5
tension[1]	26.8
tired sleepy during work or leisure time[1]	74.6
trouble falling asleep[1]	54.0
trouble waking up[1]	70.4
unsteadiness, vertigo[1]	11.3
vegetative symptoms[1]	14.1
wakes up often, trouble falling asleep again[1]	118.0
waking up to early[1]	59.2

Broadwell, Darcey, Hudnell, et al (1995)
n = 32
Diagnostic Criteria:
Gender: 15/17
Age: 47.6 (9.0)
Race: 11/3/17/1/0/0

Population Setting: micro-electronic factory workers
Nationality: US
Other Sample Characteristics: exposed to multiple solvents >1 year
Method of Reporting: eye exam
Timeframe: current

Symptom	%
color discrimination deficit	36

Juntunen, Metikainen, Antii-Poika, et al. (1985)
n = 31
Diagnostic Criteria:
Gender: 31/0
Age: 41.5 (8.0)
Race:

Population Setting: offset printers
Nationality: Finland
Other Sample Characteristics: tolulene exposure 22 years (7.4 years)
Method of Reporting: [1]interview; [2]neurological exam
Timeframe: current

Symptoms	%

Symptoms	%

abnormal findings in neuropsychological examinations[2]	7
cerebellar disturbances[1]	6
cerebellar signs[2]	13
cognitive disturbances[1]	13
disturbances in gait and posture[2]	9
dizziness[1]	3
headache[1]	13
insomnia[1]	6
memory disturbance[1]	19

numbness[1]	22
pains of the extremities[1]	9
peripheral nervous system symptoms[1]	25
peripheral neuropathy[2]	19
psychic disturbances[1]	13
slightly abnormal EEG findings[2]	19
tremor[2]	13

PSYCHIATRIC

Fox, Lees-Haley, Earnest, et al.
(1995)
n = 397
Diagnostic Criteria:
Gender: 165/232
Age: 37.4

Race:
Population Setting: HMO patients
Nationality: US
Other Sample Characteristics:
Method of Reporting: self report
Timeframe: 2 years

Symptoms	%
concentration	45
dizziness	30
ear ringing	22
fatigue	55
headache	52

Symptoms	%
impatience	53
irritability	55
memory	31
noise sensitivity	18
visual	21

Philips & Hunter (1982)
n = 300
Diagnostic Criteria:
Gender: [1]125/[2]175
Age: 16-60
Race:

Population Setting: psychiatric
hospital inpatients and outpatients
Nationality: UK
Other Sample Characteristics:
Method of Reporting: self report
Timeframe:

Symptoms	%
classical migraine[1]	1.7
classical migraine[2]	4.0

Symptoms	%
common migraine[1]	5.7
common migraine[2]	7.7

mixed headache[1]	1.3
mixed headache[2]	7.3

tension headache[1]	26.0
tension headache[2]	31.7

Rothenberg (1986)
n = 12
Diagnostic Criteria:
Gender: 6/6
Age: 16-60
Race:

Population Setting: psychiatric
inpatients
Nationality:
Other Sample Characteristics:
Method of Reporting: observation
Timeframe: current

Symptom	%
amenorrhea	0.0
binge-eating	0.0
disturbance of body image	16.7
eating & food rituals	16.7
excessive cleanliness	0.0
excessive orderliness	8.3
intense fear of becoming obese	0.0
laxative & diuretic abuse	0.0
miserliness	0.0
no known physical illness accounting for weight loss	100.0
perfectionism	25.0

Symptom	%
refusal to maintain normal weight	8.3
rigidity & fear of change	58.3
rumination on food & calories	8.3
sadistic toward own body	50.0
scrupulousness & self-righteousness	33.3
self-induced vomiting	8.3
weight loss of at least 25% of original body weight	8.3

Newmark, Raft, Toomey, et al.
(1975)
n = 160
Diagnostic Criteria:
Gender:
Age:
Race:

Population Setting: university
hospital psychiatric clinic inpatients
and outpatients
Nationality: US
Other Sample Characteristics:
Method of Reporting: rater report
Timeframe: current

Symptoms	%
agitation	18
ambivalence	47
amnesia	4
anxiety	70

Symptoms	%
archaic or magical thinking	2
autism	7
blocking	7

circumstantial	6
concrete thinking	6
confabulation	2
delusions	11
depersonalization	3
depression	78
disorientation to person	3
disorientation to place	12
disorientation to time	9
echolalia	0
echopraxia	0
flat affect	34
hallucinations	7
inappropriate affect	21
incoherent	9
labile	19
loose association	8
loss of ego boundaries	5

mutism	1
negativism	4
neologisms	0
oneiric state	0
overinclusion	7
paleologic thinking	1
paralogia	5
perseveration	7
regression	9
retardation of speech	6
sensitivity	31
social withdrawal	32
stereotyped behavior	6
stilted language	1
symbolism	2
tangential	11
variability	17
verbigeration	0

Control Groups: Child and Adolescent

CLINIC-REFERRED CHILDREN

Landau & Milichiwidiger (1991)
n = 76
Diagnostic Criteria:
Gender: 76/0
Age: 11.9 (1.7)
Race:
Population Setting: outpatient child
psychiatry clinic

Nationality: US
Other Sample Characteristics: clinic
referred for academic, behavioral,
psychiatric disorder
Method of Reporting: self-report
Timeframe: current

Symptom	%
can't attend to fun activities	28
can't sit still	47
change activities without finishing	22
doesn't finish schoolwork	25
doesn't listen in school	24
doesn't pay attention	30
leaves games unfinished	16
leaves meals/TV before finished	7
lose books and papers	20
parents must repeat commands	37
parents yell-don't know why	36

Symptom	%
push ahead in line/ can't wait turn	9
rush about without thinking	28
rush through school assignments	28
talk at school when shouldn't	28
teacher complains out of seat	16
teacher must repeat instructions	28
trouble attending school	30
trouble finding things	18

Frick, et al. (1994)
n = 440
Diagnostic Criteria:
Gender: 336/104
Age: 9.5 (4-17)
Race: 268/88/66/7/0/9
Population Setting: mental health
clinic

Nationality: US
Other Sample Characteristics: clinic
referred for behavioral problems
Method of Reporting: parent or
teacher-report
Timeframe: current

Symptom	%
angry	32
animal	12
annoy	38
argue	55
blame	38
break	12
bully	18
con	19
cruel	5
dark	8
defy	50
fights	27
fires	3

Symptoms	%
lie	31
mug	10
rape	5
ridicule	47
run	8
spiteful	22
steal	34
taunts	13
temper	48
touchy	34
truant	6
vandal	17
weapon	11

DELINQUENTS

Chiles, Miller, & Cox (1980)
n = 92
Diagnostic Criteria:
Gender: 74/18
Age: 13.9
Race: 24/0/0/0/0/4

Population Setting: adolescent
correctional facility
Nationality: US
Other Sample Characteristics:
Method of Reporting: structured
interview
Timeframe:

Symptom	%
arson	14.1
difficulty concentrating	19.5
diminished interest in activities	29.3
discouraged	21.1
dysphoric mood	31.9
eat less	30
eat more	25.3
encopresis	4.3
enuresis	27.5
excessive guilt	24.4
feeling like a failure	18.7
fighting frequently	14.3
frequent lying	48.4
frequently breaks rules	50.5
gained weight	40.2

Symptoms	%
hypersomnia	12.1
indecision	12
insomnia	34.1
less energy, fatigue	27.2
lost weight	33.7
psychomotor agitation	21.7
psychomotor retardation	12
runaway	61.5
self-reproach	35.1
short attention span	34.8
stealing	34.5
suicide attempt	10
suicide ideation	23
tease children-animals	15.2
unable to sit still	42

used a weapon (gun, knife, club)	28.6
vandalism	53.8
wanting punishment	18.9

wants to be alone	18.7
wants to be with people	32.6

ELEMENTARY SCHOOL CHILDREN

Waldman & Lilienfeld (1991)
n = 105
Diagnostic Criteria:
Gender: 105/0
Age: 8-12

Population Setting: public and
parochial elementary schools
Nationality: Canada
Other Sample Characteristics:
Method of Reporting: teacher report
Timeframe: current

Symptom	%
actively defies	19
angry/resents	22
annoys	28
blames others	28
blurts answers	23
bullies	19
difficulty playing quietly	32
difficulty remaining seated	26
difficulty sustaining	43
difficulty waiting turn	22
doesn't listen	39
easily distracted	49
fails to finish chores	43

Symptom	%
fidgets	36
interrupts	25
loses temper	21
loses things	35
messy/sloppy	37
often argues	17
often talks	34
physically dangerous	16
shifts activities	38
spiteful	15
swears	13
touchy	25

HIGH SCHOOL STUDENTS

Carter & Duncan (1984)
n = 421
Diagnostic Criteria:
Gender: 0/421
Age:
Race:

Population: rural high school students
Nationality: US
Other Sample Characteristics:
Method of Reporting: self-report
Timeframe: current

Symptom	%
self-induced vomiting	9

PSYCHIATRIC-REFERRED CHILDREN

Milich, Widiger, & Landau (1987)
n = 76
Diagnostic Criteria:
Gender: 76/0
Age: 11.9 (1.7)
Race:

Population Setting: child-psychiatry
outpatient clinic
Nationality: US
Other Sample Characteristics:
Method of Reporting: parent
interview
Timeframe:

Symptom	%
acts w/out thinking	61
breaking in	11
can't concentrate	70
can't sit still	25
cruelty to animals	1
destroys property	13
doesn't listen	66
doesn't take turns	51
easily distracted	80
fails to finish	63
games unfinished	28
hooky	7
hurt someone	3
interrupts a lot	58

Symptom	%
lies	25
needs supervision	58
on the go	51
restless sleeper	17
runaway	3
runs around	26
runs, climbs	32
sets fires	12
shifts activities	51
steals	14
suspended	14
unorganized	58
used knife or gun	11

SECONDARY SCHOOL STUDENTS

Choquet, Menke, & Ledoux (1989)
n = 327
Diagnostic Criteria:
Gender: [1]173/[2]154
Age:
Race:

Population Setting: state and private
secondary schools
Nationality: France
Other Sample Characteristics:
Method of Reporting: self-report
Timeframe: lifetime

Symptom	%
doesn't drink[1]	12.7
doesn't drink[2]	35.7

Symptoms	%
drinks infrequently[1]	20.2
drinks infrequently[2]	27.9

drinks regularly[1]	48.6
drinks regularly[2]	11.0

drinks weekly[1]	16.8
drinks weekly[2]	24.7

SPECIAL EDUCATION STUDENTS

Pelham, Evans, & Gnagy (1992)
$\underline{n}$ = 364
Diagnostic Criteria:
Gender: 364/0
Age: 5-19
Race:

Population Setting: special education classroom students
Nationality: US
Other Sample Characteristics:
Method of Reporting: teacher report
Timeframe: current

Symptom	%
actively defies or refuses adult requests/rules	30
angry or resentful	26
argues w/adults	28
blames other for own mistakes	34
blurts out answers before questions completed	37
deliberately does things that annoy others	27
difficulty following through on instructions from others	52
difficulty playing quietly	27
difficulty sustaining attention in tasks or play	50
does not seem to listen	53
fidgets w/hands or feet or squirms in seat	50
has difficulty awaiting turn	29

Symptom	%
has difficulty remaining seated	34
interrupts or intrudes on others	31
is easily distracted	63
often engages in dangerous activities w/out considering consequences	21
often loses temper	23
often loses things necessary for tasks or activities	43
often talks excessively	43
shifts from one uncompleted activity to another	43
spiteful or vindictive	14
swears or uses obscene language	14
touch or easily annoyed by others	31

Control Groups: Elderly

ALZEIMER'S DISEASE SPOUSES

Patterson, et al. (1990)
n = 21
Diagnostic Criteria:
Gender:
Age: 70.0 (5.64, 59-79)
Race:

Population Setting: community
Nationality: US
Other Sample Characteristics:
Method of Reporting: interviewer rating
Timeframe: 1 week

Symptom	%
agitation	5
anxiety	35
appetite loss	0
behavioral disturbance	14
cyclic functions	43
difficulty falling asleep	19
diurnal variation	5
early-morning awakenings	19
ideational disturbance	19
irritability	48
lack of energy	10
lack of reactivity	10
loss of interest	0

Symptom	%
mood-congruent delusions	0
mood-related signs	86
multiple awakenings	25
multiple physical complaints	10
pessimism	14
physical signs	14
poor self-esteem	19
retardation	5
sadness	67
suicide	5
weight loss	10

FRAIL ELDERLY

Mui (1993)
n = 1272
Diagnostic Criteria:
Gender: 373/899
Age: 65+
Race: 0/1272/0/0/0/0

Population Setting: National long term care channeling demonstration subjects
Nationality: US
Other Sample Characteristics:
Method of Reporting: self-report
Timeframe: 1 week

Symptom	%
concentration problems	35.3
constantly tired	51
crying spells	28.7

Symptoms	%
feeling depressed	43.9
feeling lonely	53.4
poor appetite	22.1

shortness of breath	30.2
sleep problems	42.9

Mui (1993)
n = 211
Diagnostic Criteria:
Gender: 65/146
Age: 65+
Race: 0/0/211/0/0/0

Population Setting: National long
term care
channelling demostration subjects
Nationality: US
Other Sample Characteristics:
Method of Reporting: self-report
Timeframe: 1 week

Symptom	%
concentration problems	45.7
constantly tired	61.2
crying spells	40.7
feeling depressed	61.0

Symptom	%
feeling lonely	71.3
poor appetite	41.2
shortness of breath	44.5
sleep problems	50.4

NURSING HOME

Chandler & Chandler (1988)
n = 65
Diagnostic Criteria:
Gender: 15/50
Age: 80.2 (28-103)
Race:

Population Setting: nursing home
residents
Nationality: US
Other Sample Characteristics:
Method of Reporting: chart review
Timeframe: during nursing home stay

Symptom	%
aggressive outbursts (mild)	12
aggressive outbursts (severe)	3
agitation (mild)	15

Symptom	%
agitation (severe)	17
anxiety/depression	12
confabulation	3

Zimmer, Watson, Treat (1984)
n = 1139
Diagnostic Criteria:
Gender:
Age:
Race:

Population Setting: nursing home
patients
Nationality: US
Other Sample Characteristics:
Method of Reporting: medical
records
Timeframe:

Symptoms	%
dangerous ambulation	5.4
hoarding	0.6
inappropriate ambulation	3.8
inappropriate urination/ defecation	1.0
indirectly endangering others	0.4
physical self-abuse	4.3
physically aggressive	8.3
physically disruptive	2.5

Symptoms	%
physically resistive to care	11.4
reclusive	5.0
sexually disturbing	0.4
taking others' belongings and food	1.1
verbally disruptive	12.6

Cohen-Mansfield (1986)
n = 66
Diagnostic Criteria:
Gender: 15/51
Age: 83.9 (59-96)
Race:
Population Setting: nursing home residents

Nationality: US
Other Sample Characteristics:
Symptoms occurring at least once a day
Method of Reporting: rater report
Timeframe: current

Symptom	%
biting	3.0
complaining/negativism	32.5
constant unwaranted request for attention or help	53.0
cursing or verbal aggression	36.8
general restlessness	47.5
hitting/kicking	21.2
hurting self or other with cigarette	0.0
inappropriate dressing or disrobing	19.7
making strange noises/screaming	10.8
pacing, aimless wandering	37.8

Symptom	%
spitting	12.1
throwing things	3.0
try to get to different place	5.0

References

Ackerman, P.T., Dykman, R. A., & Peters, J. E. (1977). Teenage status of hyperactive and nonhyperactive learning disabled boys. *American Journal of Orthopsychiatry, 47(4)*, 577-596.

Albert, N. & Beck, A. T. (1975). Incidence of depression in earlyadolescence: A preliminary study. *Journal of Youth and Adolescence, 4(4)*, 301-307.

Aldrich, M. S., & Chauncey, J. B. (1990). Are morning headaches partof obstructive sleep apnea syndrome. *Archives of Internal Medicine, 150,* 1265-1267.

Amodei, N., Elkin, B. B., Burge, S. K., Rodriguez-Andrew, S., Lane,P., & Seale, J. P. (1994). Psychiatric problems experienced by primary care patients who misuse alcohol. *The International Journal of the Addictions, 29(5)*, 609-626.

Ardila, A. & Bateman, J. R. (1995). Psychoactive substance use: Some associated characteristics. *Addictive Behaviors, 20(4),* 549-554.

Becker, J. T., Boller, F., Lopez, O. L., Saxton, J., & McGonigle, K. L. (1994). The natural history of Alzheimer's disease: Description of study cohort and accuracy of diagnosis. *Archives of Neurology, 51,* 585-594.

Bjornsson, E., Plaschke, P., Norrman, E., Janson, C., Lundback, B., Rosenhall, A., Lindholm, N., Rosenhall, L., Berglund, E., & Boman, G. (1994). Symptoms related to asthma and chronic bronchitis in three areas of Sweeden. *European Respiratory Journal, 7,* 2146-2153.

Blakely, A. A., Howard, R. C., Sosich, R. M., Murdoch, J. C., Menkes, D. B., & Spears, G. F. S. (1991). Psychiatric symptoms, personality and ways of coping in chronic fatigue syndrome. *Pyschological Medicine, 21,* 347-362.

Blau, J. N. & Solomon, F. (1985). Smell and other sensory disturbances in migraine. *Journal of Neurology, 232,* 275-276.

Bowler, R., Huel, G., Mergler, D., Cone, J., Rauch, S., & Hartney, C. (1996). Symptom base rates after chemical exposrue for White, Hispanic, and African-Americans. *Neurotoxicology, 17.*Bowling, A. (1990). The prevalence of psychiatric morbidity among people aged 85 and over living at home: Associations with reported somatic symptoms and with consulting behaviour. *Social Psychiatry and Psychiatric Epidemiology, 25,* 132-140.

Breslau, N. (1992). Migraine, suicidal ideation, and suicide attempts*Neurology, 42,* 392-395.

Breslau, N., Davis, G. C., & Andreski, P. (1991). Migraine, psychiatric disorders, and suicide attempts: An epidemiologic study of young adults. *Psychiatry Research, 37 (1),* 11-23.

Breslau, N., Roth, T., Rosenthal, L., & Andreski, P. (1996). Sleepdisturbance and psychiatric disorders: A longitudinal epidemiological study of young adults. *Biological Psychiatry, 39,* 411-418.

Broadwell, D. K., Darcey, D. J., Hudnell, H. K., Otto, D. A., & Boyes,W. K. (1995). Work-site clinical and neurobehavioral assessment of solvent-exposed microelectronics workers. *American Journal of Industrial Medicine, 27,* 677-698.

Bulpitt, C. J., Dollery, C. T., & Hoffbrand, B. I. (1974). A symptom questionnaire for hypertensive patients. *Journal of Chronic Disease, 27,* 309-323.

Carlson G. A., & Kashani, J. H. (1988). Manic symptoms in a non-referred adolescent population. *Journal of Affective Disorders, 15,* 219-226.

Carter, J. A. & Duncan, P. A. (1984). Binge-eating and vomiting: A survey of a high school population. *Psychology in the Schools, 21,* 198-203.

Chandler, J. D. & Chandler, J. E. (1988). The prevalence of neuropsychiatric disorders in a nursing home population. *Journal of Geriatric Psychiatry and Neurology, 1,* 71-76.

Chee, K. Y. & Sachdev, P. (1997). A controlled study of sensory tics in Gilles de la Tourette syndrome and obsessive-compulsive disorder using a structured interview. *Journal of Neurology, Neurosurgery, and Psychiatry, 62,* 188-192.

Chiles, A., Miller, M. L., & Cox, G. B. (1980). Depression in an adolescent delinquent population. *Archives of General Psychiatry, 37,* 1179-1184.

Choquet, M. (1989).The body image of suicidal adolescents: An epidemiological approach. *Psychologie Medicale, 21(4),* 449-452. Cirignotta, F., D'Alessandro, R., Partinen, M., Zucconi, M., Cristina E., Gerardi, R., Cacciatore, F. M., & Lugaresi, E. (1989). Prevalence of every night snoring and obstructive sleep apnoeas among 30-69-year-old men in Bologna, Italy. *Acta Psychiatrica Scandinavica, 79,* 366-372.

Clifford, R. D., Radford, M., Howell, J. B., & Holgate, S. T. (1989). Prevalence of respiratory symptoms among 7 and 11 year old schoolchildren and association with asthma. *Archives of Disease in Childhood, 64,* 1118-1125.

Cohen-Mansfield, J. (1986). Agitated behaviors in the elderly: II. Preliminary results in the cognitively deteriorated. *Journal of the American Geriatric Society, 34(10),* 722-727.

Cottler, L. B., Compton, W. M., III, Mager, D., Spitznagel, E. L., & Janca, A. (1992). Posttraumatic stress disorder among substance users from the general population. *American Journal of Psychiatry, 149(5),* 664-670.

Cuijpers, C. E. J., Wesseling, G. J., Swaen, G. M. H., Sturmans, F., & Wouters, E. F. M. (1994). Asthma-related symptoms and lung function in primary school children. *Journal of Asthma, 31(4),* 301-312.

Demallie, D., Cottler, L. B., & Compton, W. M. (1995). Alcohol abuse and dependence: Consistency in reporting of symptoms over ten years. *Addiction, 90(5),* 615-625.

De Smet, Y., Ruberg, M., Serdaru, M., Dubois, B., Lhermitte, F., & Agid, Y. (1982). Confusion, dementia and anticholinergics in Parkinson's disease. *Journal of Neurology, Neurosurgery, and Psychiatry, 45,* 1161-1164.

Degonda, M., Wyss, M., & Angst, J. (1993). The Zurich Study: XVIII.Obsessive-compulsive disorders and syndromes in the general population. *European Archives of Psychiatry and Clinical Neuroscience, 243,* 16-22.

Dick, C. L., Bland, R. C., & Newman, S. C. (1994). Panic disorder. *Acta Psychiatrica Scandinavica Suppement, 376,* 45-53.

Doull, I. J., Williams, A. A., Freezer, N. J., & Holgate, S. T. (1996).Descriptive study of cough, wheeze and school absence in childhood. *Thorax, 51,* 630-631.

Droller, H. & Pemberton, J. (1953). Vertigo in a random sample of elderly people living in their homes. *Journal of Laryngology and Otology, 67(11),* 689-695.

Duncan, D. & Snow, W. G. (1987). Base rates in neuropsychology.*Professional Psychology: Research and Practice, 18,* 368-370.

Enright, P. L., Kronmal, R. A., Higgins, M. W., Schenker, M. B., & Haponik, E. F. (1994). Prevalence and correlates of respiratory symptoms and disease in the elderly. *Chest, 106(3),* 827-834.

Escobar, J. I., Burnam, M. A., Karno, M., Forsythe, A., & Golding, J.M. (1987). Somatization in the community. *Archives of General Psychiatry, 44,* 713-718.

Fava, M., Rosenbaum, J. F., Pava, J. A., McCarthy, M. K., Steingard, R. J., & Bouffides, E. (1991). Anger attacks in depressed outpatients and their response to fluoxetine. *Psychopharmacology Bulletin, 27(3),* 275-279.

Fernandez, E. & Sheffield, J. (1996). Descriptive features and causalattributions of headache in an Australian community. *Headache, 36,* 246-250.

Fitzpatrick, M. F., Martin, K., Fossey, E., Shapiro, C. M., Elton, R. A.,& Douglas, N. J. (1993). Snoring, asthma and sleep disturbance in Britain: A community-based survey. *European Respiratory Journal, 6,* 531-535.

Flament, M. F., Koby, E., Rapoport, J. L., Berg, C. J., Zahn, T., Cox,C., Denckla, M. & Lenane, M. (1990). Childhood obsessive-compulsive disorder: A prospective follow-up study. *Journal of Child Psychology and Psychiatry, 31(3),* 363-380.

Forero, R., Bauman, A., Young, L., Booth, M. & Nutbeam, D. (1996). Asthma, health behaviors, social adjustment, and psychosomatic symptoms in adolescence. *Journal of Asthma, 33(3),* 157-164.

Fox, D., Lees-Haley, P., Earnest, K., & Dolezal-Wood, S. (1995). Base rates of postconcussive symptoms in health maintenance organization patients and controls. *Neuropsychology, 9(4),* 606-611.

Fox, D., Lees-Haley, P., Earnest, K., & Dolezal-Wood, S. (1995). Post-concussive symptoms: Base rates and etiology in psychiatric patients. The Clinical *Neuropsychologist, 9(1),* 89-92.

Freeston, M. H., Dugas, M. J., Letarte, H., Rhéaume, J., Blais, F., & Ladouceur, R. (1996). Physical symptoms associated with worry in a nonclinical population. *Journal of Anxiety Disorders, 10(5),* 365-377.

Frick, P. J., Lahey, B. B., Applegate, B., Kerdyck, L., Ollendick, T., Hynd, G. W., Garfinkel, B., Greenhill, L., Biederman, J., Barkley, R. A. et al. (1994). DSM-IV field trials for the disruptive behavior disorders: Symptom utility estimates. *Journal of the American Academy of Child and Adolescent Psychiatry, 33(4),* 529-539.

Friedman, A. (1994). Old-onset Parkinson's disease compared with young-onset disease: Clinical differences and similarities. *Acta Neurologica Scandinavica, 89,* 258-261.

Frost, R. O., Krause, M. S., & Steketee, G. (1995). The relationship of the Yale-Brown Obsessive Compulsive Scale (YBOCS) to other measures of obsessive compulsive symptoms in a nonclinical population. *Journal of Personality Assessment, 65(1),* 158-168.

Fuhrer, R. & Wessley, S. (1995). The epidemiology of fatigue and depression: A French primary-care study. *Psychological Medicine, 25,* 895-905.

Garrison, C. Z., Schluchter, M. D., Schoenbach, V. J., & Kaplan, B. K. (1989). Epidemiology of depressive symptoms in young adolescents. *Journal of the American Academy of Child and Adolescent Psychiatry, 28(3),* 343-351.

Gerbaldo, H. & Thaker, G. (1991). Photophilic and photophobicbehaviour in patients with schizophrenia and depression. *Canadian Journal of Psychiatry, 36(9),* 677-679.

Glosser, G., Wolfe, N., Kliner-Krenzel, L., & Albert, M. L. (1994). Cross-cultural cognitive examination performance in patients with Parkinson's disease and Alzheimer's disease. *The Journal of Nervous and Mental Disease, 182,* 432-436.

Gordon, N. G. (1977). Base rates and the decision making model in clinical neuropsychology. *Cortex, 13(1),* 3-10.

Gouvier, W. D. (1999). Base rates and clinical decision making in neuropsychology. In J. J. Sweet (Ed.), *Forensic neuropsychology: Fundamentals and practice.* Lisse, Netherlands: Swets & Zeitlinger.

Gouvier, W. D. (2001). Are you sure you're really telling the truth?*Neurorehabilitation, 16(4),* 215-219.

Gouvier, W.D., Cubic, B., Jones, G., Brantley, D., & Cutlip, Q. (1992). Post-concussive symptoms and daily stress in normal and head injured college populations. *Archives of Clinical Neuropsychology, 7,* 193-211.

Gouvier, W. D., Hayes, J. S., & Smiroldo, B. B. (1998). The significance of base rates, test sensitivity, test specificity, and subject's lnowledge of symptoms in assessing TBI sequelae and malingering. In C. Reynolds (Ed.), Detection of malingering during head injury litigation (pp. 55-79). New York: Plenum Press.

Gouvier, W. D., Pinkston, J. B., Maria, M. P. S., & Cherry, K. E. (2002). Base rate analysis in cross-cultural clinical psychology—diagnosis accuracy in the balance. In F. R. Ferraro (Ed.), *Minority and cross-cultural aspects of neuropsychological assessment.* Lisse, Netherlands: Swets & Zeitlinger.

Grant, I., Atkinson, J. H., Hesselink, J. R., Kennedy, C. J., Richman, D. D., Spector, S. A., & McCutchan, J. A. (1987). Evidence for early central nervous system involvement in the acquired immunodificiency syndrome (AIDS) and other human immunodeficiency virus (HIV) infections. *Annals of Internal Medicine, 107(6),* 828-836.

Hale, W. E., Perkins, L. L., May, F. E., Marks, R. G., & Stewart, R. B. (1986). Symptom prevalence in the elderly: An evaluation of age, sex, disease, and medication use. *Journal of the American Geriatrics Society, 34(5),* 333-340.

Hallman, J. (1986). The prementrual syndrome-an equivalent of depression? *Acta Psychiatrica Scandinavica, 73,* 403-411.

Hannay, D. R. (1978). Symptom prevalence in the community. *Journal of the Royal College of General Practitioners, 28,* 492-499.

Haraldsson, P. O., Carenfelt, C., & Tingvall, C. (1992). Sleep apnea syndrome symptoms and automobile driving in a general population. *Journal of Clinical Epidemiology, 45(8),* 821-825.

Hart, H., Bax, M., & Jenkins, S. (1984). Health and behaviour in preschool children. *Child: Care, Health and Development, 10,* 1-16.

Hartmann, B. W., Kirchengast, S., Albrecht, A., Metka, M., & Huber, J. C. (1995). Hysterectomy increases the symptomatology of postmenopausal syndrome. *Gynecological Endocrinology, 9(3),* 247-52.

Heaton, K. W., Ghosh, S., & Braddon, F. E. M. (1991). How bad are the symptoms and bowel dysfunction of patients with the irrtable bowel syndrome? A prospective, controlled study with empahsis on stool form. *Gut, 32,* 73-79.

Heaton, K. W., O'Donnell, L. J., Braddon, F. E., Mountford, R. A., Hughes, A. O., & Cripps, P. J. (1992). Symptoms of irritable bowel syndrome in a British urban community: Consulters and nonconsulters. *Gastroenterology, 102(6),* 1962-1967.

Heilman, K. & Valenstein (2003). Clinical Neuropsychology. New York: Oxford University Press.

Hendren, R. L., Hodde-Vargas, J., Yeo, R. A., Vargas, L. A., Brooks, W. M., & Ford, C. (1995). Neurpsychophysiological study of children at risk for schizophrenia: A preliminary report. *Journal of the American Academy of Child and Adolescent Psychiatry, 34(10),* 1284-1291.

Hill, R. A., Standen, P. J., & Tattersfield, A. E. (1989). Asthma, wheezing, and school absence in primary schools. *Archives of Disease in Childhood, 64,* 246-251.

Hinds, J. P., Eidelman, B. H., & Wald, A. (1990). Prevalence of bowel dysfunction in multiple sclerosis: A population survey. *Gastroenterology, 98(6),* 1538-1542.

Hochstrasser, B. & Angst, J. (1996). The Zurich Study: XXII. Epidemiology of gastrointestinal complaints and comorbidity with anxiety and depression. *European Archives of Psychiatry and Clinical Neuroscience, 246,* 261-272.

Hollander, E., Greenwald, S., Neville, D., Johnson, J., Hornig, C. D., & Weissman, M. M. (1996/1997). Uncomplicated and comorbid obsessive-compulsive disorder in an epidemiologic sample. *Depression and Anxiety, 4,* 111-119.

Honsberg, A. E., Dodge, R. R., Cline, M. G., & Quan, S. F. (1995). Incidence and remission of habitual snoring over a five to six-year period. *Chest, 108(3),* 604-609.

House, A., Dennis, M., Mogridge, L., Warlow, C., Hawton, K. & Jones, L. (1991). Mood disorders in the year after first stroke. *British Journal of Psychiatry, 158,* 83-92.

Huerta-Franco, M. R. & Malacara, J. M. (1993). Association of physical and emotional symptoms with the menstrual cycle and life-style. *Journal of Reproductive Medicine, 38(6),* 448-454.

Isoaho, R., Keistinen, T., Laippala, P., & Kivela, S. L. (1995). Chronic obstructive pulmonary disease and symptoms related to depression in elderly persons. *Psychological Reports, 76,* 287-297.

Jebbink, H. J. A., Bruijs, P. P. M., Bravenboer, B., Akkermans, L. M. A., vanBerge-Henegouwen, G. P. & Smout, A. J. P. M. (1994). Gastric myoelectrical activity in patients with type I diabetes mellitus and autonomic neuropathy. *Digestive Diseases and Sciences, 39(11),* 2376-2383.

Jennum, P., Hein, H. O., Suadicani, P., & Gyntelberg, F. (1994). Headache and cognitive dysfunctions in snorers. *Archives of Neurology, 51,* 937-942.

Johnson, S. K., DeLuca, J., & Natelson, B. H. (1996). Assessing somatization disorder in the chronic fatigue syndrome. *Psychosomatic Medicine, 58,* 50-57.

Jolleys, J. V. (1988). Reported prevalence of urinary incontinence in women in a general practice. *British Medical Journal (Clinical Research Ed), 296,* 1300-1302.

Judd, L. L., Rapaport, M. H., Paulus, M. P. & Brown, J. L. (1994). Subsyndromal symptomatic depression: A new mood disorder? *Journal of Clinical Psychiatry, 55(Suppl. 4),* 18-28.

Juntunen, J., Matikainen, E., Antti-Poika, M., Suroanta, H. & Valle, M. (1985). Nervous system effects of long-term occupational exposure to toluene. *Acta Neurologica Scandinavica, 72,* 512-517.

Kales, J. D., Kales, A., Bixler, E. O., Soldatos, C. R., Cadieux, R. J., Kashurba, G. J., & Vela-Bueno, A. (1984). Biopsychobehavioral correlates of insomnia, V: Clinical characteristics and behavioral correlates. *American Journal of Psychiatry, 141(11),* 1371-1376.

Kanbayashi, Y., Nakata, Y., Fujii, K., Kita, M., & Wada, K. (1994). ADHD-related behavior among non-referred children: Parents' ratings of DSM-III-R symptoms. *Child Psychiatry and Human Development, 25(1),* 13-29.

Kashani, J. H., Rosenberg, T. K., & Reid, J. C. (1989). Developmental perspectives in child and adolescent depressive symptoms in a community sample. *American Journal of Psychiatry, 146(7),* 871-875.

Katona, C., Livingston, G., Manela, M., Leek, C., Mullan, E., Orrell, M., D'Ath, P., & Zeitlin, D. (1997). The symptomatology of depression in the elderly. *International Clinical Psychopharmacology, 12(Suppl. 7),* S19-S23.

Kaye, J., Kaye, K., & Madow, L. (1983). Sleep patterns in patients with cancer and patients with cardiac disease. *Journal of Psychology, 117,* 107-113.

Khalsa, M. E., Tashkin, D. P., & Perrochet, B. (1992). Smoked cocaine: Patterns of use and pulmonary consequences. *Journal of Psychoactive Drugs, 24(3),* 265-272.

Kinjo, Y., Higashi, H., Nakano, A., Sakamoto, M., & Saka, R. (1993). Profile of subjective complaints and activities of daily living among current patients with Minamata disease after three decades. *Environmental Research, 63,* 241-251.

Kivela, S. L., Nissinen, A., Tuomilehto, J., Pekkanen, J., Punsar, S., Lammi, U. K., & Puska, P. (1986). Prevalence of depressive and other symptoms in elderly Finnish men. *Acta Psychiatrica Scandinavica, 73,* 93-100.

Kivela, S. L. & Pahkala, K. (1988). Clinician-rated symptoms and signs of depression in aged Finns. *International Journal of Social Psychiatry, 34(4),* 274-284.

Klink, M. E., Dodge, R., & Quan, S. F. (1994). The relation of sleep complaints to respiratory symptoms in a general population. *Chest, 105(1),* 151-154.

Koegel, P. & Burnam, M. A. (1988). Alcoholism among homeless adults in the inner city of Los Angeles. *Archives of General Psychiatry, 45,* 1011-1018.

Krieger, J., Petiau, C., Sforza, E., Delanoe, C., Hecht, M. T., & Chamouard, V. (1993). Nocturnal pollakiuria is a symptom of obstructive sleep apnea. *Urology International, 50,* 93-97.

Kroenke, K. & Price, R. K. (1993). Symptoms in the community: Prevalence, classification, and psychiatric comorbidity. *Archives of Internal Medicine, 153(8),* 2474-2480.

Krupp, L. B., Alvarez, L. A., LaRocca, N. G., & Scheinberg, L. C. (1988). Fatigue in multiple sclerosis. *Archives of Neurology, 45,* 435-437.

Krupp, L. B., Jandorf, L., Coyle, P. K., & Mendelson, W. B. (1993). Sleep disturbance in chronic fatigue syndrome. *Journal of Psychosomatic Research, 37(4),* 325-331.

Kuh, D. L., Wadsworth, M., & Hardy, R. (1997). Women's health in midlife: The influence of the menopause, social factors and health in earlier life. *British Journal of Obstetrics and Gynecology, 104,* 923-933.

Landau, S., Milich, R., & Widiger, T. A. (1991). Conditional probabilities of child interview symptoms in the diagnosis of attention deficit disorder. *Journal of Child Psychology and Psychiatry, 32(3),* 501-513.

Larsson, L., Lundback, B., Jonsson, A., Lindstrom, M., & Jonsson, E. (1997). Symptoms related to snoring and sleep apnoea in subjects with chronic bronchitis: Report from the Obstructive Lung Disease in Northern Sweden Study. *Respiratory Medicine, 91,* 5-12.

Lavie, P. (1981). Sleep habits and sleep distrubances in industrial workers in Israel: Main findings and some characteristics of workers complaining of excessive daytime sleepiness. *Sleep, 4(2),* 147-158.

Lavie, P. (1983). Incidence of sleep apnea in a presumably healthy working population: A significant relationship with excessive daytime sleepiness. *Sleep, 6(4),* 312-318.

Lee, K. A. &. Rittenhouse, C. A (1991). Prevalence of perimenstrual symptoms in employed women. *Women and Health, 17(3),* 17-32.

Lees-Haley, P. R. & Brown, R. S. (1993). Neuropsychological complaint base rates of 170 personal injury claimants. *Archives of Clinical Neuropsychology, 8,* 203-209.

Linet, M. S., Stewart, W. F., Celentano, D. D., Ziegler, D., & Sprecher, M. (1989). An epidemiologic study of headache among adolescents and young adults. *Journal of the American Medical Association, 261(15),* 2211-2216.

Linna, S. L., Moilanen, I., Keistinen, H., Ernvall, M. L., & Karppinen, M. M. (1991). Prevalence of psychosomatic symptoms in children. *Psychotherapy and Psychosomatics, 56,* 85-87.

Little, B. B., Snell, L. M., Rosenfeld, C. R., Gilstrap, L. C., III, & Grant, N. F. (1990). Failure to recognize fetal alcohol syndrome in newborn infants. *American Journal of Diseases of Children, 177,* 1142-1146.

Litz, B. T., Keane, T. M., Fisher, L., Marx, B., & Monaco, V. (1992). Physical health complaints in combat-related post-traumatic stress disorder: A preliminary report. *Journal of Traumatic Stress, 5(1),* 131-141.

Lundberg, I., Michelsen, H., Nise, G., Hogstedt, C., Hogberg, M., Alfredsson, L., Almkvist, O., Gustavsson, A., Hagman, M., Herlofson, J., Hindmarsh, T., & Wennberg, A. (1995). Neuropsychiatric function of housepainters with previous long-term heavy exposure to organic solvents. *Sandinavian Journal of Work and Environmental Health, 21(Suppl. 1),* 1-44.

Lydiard, R. B., Greenwald, S., Weissman, M. M., Johnson, J., Drossman, D. A., & Ballenger, J. C. (1994). Panic disorder and gastrointestinal symptoms: Findings from the NIMH epidemiologic catchment area project. *American Journal of Psychiatry, 151(1),* 64-70.

Machulda, M. M., Bergquist, T. F., Ito, V., & Chew, S. (1998). Relationship between stress, coping, and postconcussion symptoms in a healthy adult population. *Archives of Clinical Neuropsychology, 13(5),* 415-424.

Mannuzza, S., Klein, R. G., Bonagura, N., Konig, P. H., & Shenker, R. (1988). Hyperactive boys almost grown up: II. Status of subjects without a mental disorder. *Archives of General Psychiatry, 45,* 13-18.

Mathew, R. J., Weinman, M. L., & Mirabi, M. (1981). Physical symptoms of depression. *British Journal of Psychiatry, 139,* 293-296.

Matthews, K. A., Wing, R. R., Kuller, L. H., Meilahn, E. N., & Plantinga, P. (1994). Influence of the perimenopause on cardiovascular risk factors and symptoms of middle-aged healthy women. *Archives of Internal Medicine, 154,* 2349-2355.

Mavrikakis, M. E., Sfikakis, P. P., Kontoyannis, S. A., Antoniades, L. G., Kontoyannis, D. A., & Moulopoulou, D. S. (1991). Clinical and laboratory parameters in adult diabetics with and without calcific shoulder periarthritis. *Calcified Tissue International, 49,* 288-291.

McCaffrey, R. J., Palav, A., O'Bryant, S. E., & Labarge, A. S. (2003). Practitioner's guide to symptom base rates in clinical neuropsychology. Plenum: New York.

McCormick, W. C., Kukull, W. A., vanBelle, G., Bowen, J. D., Teri, L., & Larson, E. B. (1994). Symptom patterns and comorbidity in the early stages of Alzheimer's disease. *Journal of the American Geriatric Society, 42(5),* 517-521.

McKinlay, S. M. & Jefferys, M. (1974). The menopausal syndrome. *British Journal of Preventative and Social Medicine, 28,* 108-115.

McLean, A., Jr., Dikmen, S., Temkin, N., Wyler, A. R., & Gale, J. L. (1984). Psychosocial functioning at 1 month after head injury. *Neurosurgery, 14(4),* 393-399.

Meehl, P. E., & Rosen, A. (1955). Antecedent probability and the efficiency of psychometric signs, patterns, or cutting scores. *Psychological Bulletin, 52,* 194-216.

Menza, M. A. & Rosen, R. C. (1995). Sleep in Parkinson's disease: The role of depression and anxiety. *Psychosomatics, 36(3),* 262-266.

Merello, M., Sabe, L., Tenson, A., Migliorelli, R., Petracchi, M., Leiguarda, R., & Starkstein, S. (1994). Extrapyramidalism in Alzheimer's disease: Prevalence, psychiatric, and neuropsychological correlates. *Journal of Neurology, Neurosurgery, and Psychiatry, 57,* 1503-1509.

Merikangas, K. R., Angst, J., & Isler, H. (1990). Migraine and psychopathology. *Archives of General Psychiatry, 47,* 849-853.

Milich, R., Widiger, T. A., & Landau, S. (1987). Differential diagnosis of attention deficit and conduct disorders using conditional probabilities. *Journal of Consulting and Clinical Psychology, 55(5),* 762-767.

Mittenberg, W., DiGiulio, D. V., Perrin, S., & Bass, A. E. (1992). Symptoms following mild head injury: Expectation as etiology. *Journal of Neurology, Neurosurgery, and Psychiatry, 55,* 200-204.

Molander, U., Milsom, I., Ekelund, P., Mellstrom, D. (1990). An epidemiological study of urinary incontinence and related urogenital symptoms in elderly women. *Maturitas, 12,* 51-60.

Moorey, H. & Soni, S. D. (1994). Anxiety symptoms in stable chronic schizophrenics. *Journal of Mental Health, 3,* 257-262.

Mui, A. C. (1993). Self-reported depressive symptoms among black and Hispanic frail elders: A sociocultural perspective. *Journal of Applied Gerontology, 12(2),* 170-187.

Muller, A., Montoya, P., Schandry, R., & Hartl, L. (1994). Changes in physical symptoms, blood pressure and quality of life over 30 days. *Behaviour Research and Therapy, 32(6),* 593-603.

Neugarten, B. L. & R. J. Kraines (1965). Menopausal symptoms in women of various ages. *Psychosomatic Medicine, 27(3),* 266-273.

Newland, C. A., Illis, L. S., Robinson, P. K., Batchelor, B. G., & Waters, W. E. (1978). A survey of headache in an English city. *Research and Clinical Studies in Headache, 5,* 1-20.

Newmark, C. S., Raft, D., Toomey, T., Hunter, W., & Mazzaglia, J. (1975). Diagnosis of schizophrenia: Pathognomonic signs or symptom clusters. *Comprehensive Psychiatry, 16(2),* 155-163.

Ng, T. P., Lim, L. C. C., & Win, K. K. (1992). An investigation of solvent-induced neuro-psychiatric disorders in spray painters. *Annals of the Academy of Medicine, 21(6),* 797-803.

Ninomiya, T., Ohmori, H., Hashimoto, K., Tsuruta, K., & Ekino, S. (1995). Expansion of methylmercury poisoning outside of Minamata: An epidemiological study on chronic methylmercury poisoning outside of Minamata. *Environmental Research, 70,* 47-50.

Norton, G. R. Harrison, B., Hauch, J. & Rhodes, L. (1985). Characteristics of people with infrequent panic attacks. *Journal of Abnormal Psychology, 94(2),* 216-221.

Noyes, R., Jr., Cook, B., Garvey, M., & Sumers, R. (1990). Reduction of gastrointestinal symptoms following treatment for panic disorder. *Psychosomatics, 31(1),* 75-79.

Nyhlin, H., Ford, M. J., Eastwood, J., Smith, J. H., Nicol, E. F., Elton, R. A., & Eastwood, M. A. (1993). Non-alimentary aspects of the irritable bowel syndrome. *Journal of Psychosomatic Research, 37(2),* 155-162.

O'Keefe, E. A., Talley, N. J., Zinsmeister, A. R., Jacobsen, S. J. (1995). Bowel disorders impair functional status and quality of life in the elderly: A population-based study. *Journal of Gerontology: Medical Sciences, 50A(4),* M184-M189.

Ohayon, M. M., Guilleminault, C., Priest, R. G., & Caulet, M. (1997). Snoring and breathing pauses during sleep: Telephone interview survey of a United Kingdom population sample. *British Medical Journal, 314,* 860-863.

Orbaek, P., Risberg, J., Rosen, I., Haeger-Aronson, B., Hagstadius, S., Hjortsberg, U., Regnell, G., Rehnstrom, S., Svensson, K., & Welinder, H. (1985). Effects of long-term exposure to solvents in the paint industry: A cross-sectional epidemiologic study with clinical and laboratory methods. *Scandinavian Journal of Work and Environmental Health, 11(Suppl. 2),* 1-28.

Patterson, M. B., Schnell, A. H., Martin, R. J., Mendez, M. F., Smyth, K. A., & Whitehouse, P. J. (1990). Assessment of behavioral and affective symptoms in Alzheimer's disease. *Journal of Geriatric Psychiatry and Neurology, 3,* 21-30.

Peckham, C. & Butler, N. (1978). A national study of asthma in childhood. *Journal of Epidemiology and Community Health, 32,* 79-85.

Pelham, W. E., Jr., Gnagy, E. M., Greenslade, K. E., & Milich, R. (1992). Teacher ratings of DSM-III-R symptoms for the disruptive behavior disorders: Prevalence, factor analyses, and conditional probabilities in a special education sample. *School Psychology Review, 21(2),* 285-299.

Pfeffer, C., Zuckerman, S., Plutchik, R., Mizruchi, M. S. (1984). Suicidal behavior in normal school children: A comparison with child psychiatric inpatients. *Journal of the American Academy of Child Psychiatry, 23 (4),* 416-423.

Pham, K. T., Grisso, J. A., & Freeman, E. W. (1997). Ovarian aging and hormone replacement therapy: Hormonal levels, symptoms, and attitudes of African-American and white women. *Journal of General and Internal Medicine, 12,* 230-236.

Philips, C. & Hunter, M. (1982). Headache in a psychiatric population. *Journal of Nervous and Mental Disease, 170(1),* 34-40.

Porter, M., Penney, G. C., Russell, D., Russell, E., & Templeton, A. (1996). A population based survey of women's experience of the menopause. *British Journal of Obstetrics and Gynaecology, 103,* 1025-1028.

Price, R. K., North, C. S., Wessely, S., & Fraser, V.J. (1992). Estimating the prevalence of chronic fatigue syndrome and associated symptoms in the community. *Public Health Reports, 107,* 514-522.

Raja, S. N., Feehan, M., Stanton, W. R., & McGee, R. (1992). Prevalence and correlates of the premenstrual syndrome in adolescence. *Journal of the American Academy of Child and Adolescent Psychiatry, 31(5),* 783-789.

Ramcharan, S., Love, E. J., Fick, G. H., & Goldfien, A. (1992). The epidemiology of premenstrual symptoms in a population-based sample of 2650 urban women: Atrributable risk and risk factors. *Journal of Clinical Epidemiology, 45(4),* 377-392.

Rasmussen, B. K., Jensen, R.. Schroll, M., & Oleson, J. (1992). Interrelations between migraine and tension-type headache in the general population. *Archives of Neurology, 49,* 914-918.

Rasmussen, B. K. & Olesen, J. (1992). Symptomatic andnonsymptomatic headaches in a general population. *Neurology, 42,* 1225-1231.

Roberts, R. E., Lewinsohn, P. M., & Seeley, J. R. (1995). Symptoms of DSM-III-R major depression in adolescence: Evidence from a epidemiological survey. *Journal of the American Academy of Child and Adolescent Psychiatry, 34(12),* 1608-1617.

Roberts, V. J., Ingram, S. M., Lamar, M., & Green, R. C. (1996). Prosody impairment and associated affective and behavioral disturbances in Alzheimer's disease. *Neurology, 47,* 1482-1488.

Rothenberg, A. (1986). Eating disorder as a modern obsessive-compulsive syndrome. *Psychiatry, 49,* 45-53.

Rubin, E. H., Morris, J. C., & Berg, L. (1987). The progression of personality changes in senile dementia of the Alzheimer's type. *Journal of the American Geriatric Society, 35(8),* 721-725.

Rubin, E. H., Morris, J. C., Storandt, M., & Berg, L. (1987). Behavioral changes in patients with mild senile dementia of the Alzheimer's type. *Psychiatry Research, 21,* 55-62.

Rutter, M., Graham, P., Chadwick, O. F., & Yule, W. (1976). Adolescent turmoil: Fact or fiction? *Journal of Child Psychology and Psychiatry, 17,* 35-56.

Saykin, A. J., Janssen, R. S., Sprehn, G. C., Kaplan, J., Spira, T. J., & O'Connor, B. (1991). Longitudinal evaluation of neuropsychological function in homosexual men with HIV infection: 18-month follow-up. *Journal of Neuropsychiatry and Clinical Neurosciences, 3(3),* 286-298.

Schaughency, E., McGee, R., Raja, S. N., Freehan, M., & Silva, P. A. (1994). Self-reported inattention, inpulsivity, and hyperactivity at ages 15 and 18 years in the general population. *Journal of the American Academy of Child and Adolesecent Psychiatry, 33(2),* 173-184.

Schoenbach, V. J., Kaplan, B. H., Grimson, R. C., & Wagner, E. H. (1982). Use of a symptom scale to study the prevalence of a depressive syndrome in young adolescents. *American Journal of Epidemiology, 116(5)*, 791-800.

Schoenbach, V. J., Kaplan, B. H., Wagner, E. H., Grimson, R. C., & Miller, F. T. Prevalence of self-reported depressive symptoms in young adolescents. *American Journal of Public Health, 73(11)*, 1281-1287.

Schvarcz, E., Palmer, M., Inberg, C. M., Aman, J., & Berne, C. (1996). Increased prevalence of upper gastrointestinal symptoms in long-term type 1 diabetes mellitus. *Diabetic Medicine*, 478-481.

Schwab, J. J., Fennell, E. B., & Warheit, G. J. (1974). The epidemiology of psychosomatic disorders. *Psychosomatics, 15*, 88-93.

Sillanpaa, M. (1992). Epilepsy in children: Prevalence, disability, and handicap. *Epilepsia, 33(3)*, 444-449.

Silverman, K., Evans, S. M., Strain, E. C., & Griffiths, R. R. (1992). Withdrawal syndrome after the double-blind cessation of caffeine consumption. *New England Journal of Medicine, 327(16)*, 1109-1114.

Sloane, P., Blazer, D., & George, L. K. (1989). Dizziness in a community elderly population. *Journal of the American Geriatrics Society, 37(2)*, 101-108.

Steinhausen, H., Nestler, V., & Spohr, H. (1982). Development and psychopathology of children with the fetal alcohol syndrome. *Developmental and Behavioral Pediatrics, 3(2)*, 49-54.

Sternbach, R. A. (1986). Survey of pain in the United States: The Nuprin Pain Report. *Clinical Journal of Pain, 2(1)*, 49-53.

Sternfeld, B., Stang, P., & Sidney, S. (1995). Relationship of migraine headaches to experience of chest pain and subsequent risk for myocardial infarction. *Neurology, 45*, 2135-2142.

Suris, J. C., Parera, N., & Puig, C. (1996). Chronic illness and emotional distress in adolescence. *Journal of Adolescent Health, 19(2)*, 153-156.

Svensson, H. O., Andersson, G. B. J., Hagstad, A., & Jansson, P. O. (1990). The relationship of low-back pain to pregnancy and gynecologic factors. *Spine, 15(5)*, 371-375.

Talley, N. J., Fett, S. L., Zinsmeister, A. R., & Melton, L. J., III. (1994). Gastrointestinal tract symptoms and self-reported abuse: A population-based study. *Gastroenterology, 107(4)*, 1040-1049.

Talley, N. J., O'Keefe, E. A., Zinsmeister, A. R., & Melton, L. J., III. (1992). Prevalence of gastrointestinal symptoms in the elderly: A population-based study. *Gastroenterology, 102(3)*, 895-901.

Talley, N. J., Zinsmeister, A. R., Schleck, C. D., & Melton, L. J., III. (1992). Dyspepsia and dyspepsia subgroups: A population-based study. *Gastroenterology, 102(4)*, 1259-1268.

Tashkin, D. P., Coulson, A. H., Clark, V. A., Simmons, M., Bourque, L. B., Duann, S., Spivey, G. H., & Gong, H. (1987), Respiratory symptoms and lung function in habitual, heavy smokers of marijuana alone, smokers of marijuana and tobacco, smokers of tobacco alone and nonsmokers. *American Review of Respiratory Disorders, 135,* 209-216.

Thomsen, P. H. (1993). Obsessive-compulsive disorder in children and adolescents: Self-reported obsessive-compulsive behaviour in pupils in Denmark. *Acta Psychiatrica Scandinavica, 88,* 212-217.

Toole, J. F., Lefkowitz, D. S., Chambless, L. E., Wijnberg, L., Paton, C. C., & Heiss, G. (1996). Self-reported transient ischemic attack and stroke symptoms: Methods and baseline prevalence. *American Journal of Epidemiology, 144(9),* 849-856.

Tse, M., Cooper, C., Bridges-Webb, C., & Bauman, A. (1993). Asthma in general practice: Opportunities for recognition and management. *Australian Family Physician, 22(5),* 736-741.

Valleni-Basile, L. A., Garrison, C. Z., Jackson, K. L., Waller, J. L., McKeown, R. E., Addy, C. L., & Cuffe, S. P. (1994). Frequency of obsessive-compulsive disorder in a community sample of young adolescents. *Journal of the American Academy of Child and Adolesecent Psychiatry, 33(6),* 782-791.

Vetter, N. J., Jones, D. A., & Victor, C. R. (1981). Urinary incontinence in the elderly at home. *Lancet,* 1275-1277.

Waite, L. M., Broe, G. A., Creasey, H., Grayson, D. A., Cullen, J. S., O'Toole, B., Edelbrock, D., & Dobson, M. (1997). Neurodegenerative and other chronic disorders among people aged 75 years and over in the community. *Medical Journal of Australia, 167,* 429-432.

Waldman, I. D. & Lilienfeld, S. O. (1991). Diagnostic efficiency of symptoms for oppositional defiant disorders and attention-deficit hyperactivity disorder. *Journal of Consulting and Clinical Psychology, 59(5),* 732-738.

Warner, P., & Bancroft, J. (1990). Factors related to self-reporting of the pre-menstrual syndrome. *British Journal of Psychiatry, 157,* 249-260.

Watkins, P. C., Williamson, D. A., & Falkowski, C. (1989). Prospective assessment of late-luteal phase dysphoric disorder.

Journal of Psychopathology and Behavioral Assessment, 11(3), 249-259.

Weiss, G., Minde, K., Werry, J. S., Douglas, V., & Nemeth, E. (1971). Studies on the hyperactive child: VIII. Five-year follow-up. *Archives of General Psychiatry, 24,* 409-414.

Weissman, M. M., Klerman, G. L., Markowitz, J. S., & Ouellette, R. (1989). Suicidal ideation and suicide attempts in panic disorder and attacks. *New England Journal of Medicine, 321(18),* 1209-1214.

Wessely, S., Chalder, T., Hirsch, S., Wallace, P., & Wright, D. (1996). Psychological symptoms, somatic symptoms, and psychiatric disorder in chronic fatigue and chronic fatigue syndrome: A prospective study in the primary care setting. *American Journal of Psychiatry, 153(8),* 1050-1059.

Wheatly, D., Balter, M., Levine, J., Lipman, R., Bauer, M., & Bonato, R. (1975). Psychiatric aspects of hypertension. *British Journal of Psychiatry, 127,* 327-336.

Wicki, W., Angst, J., & Merikangas, K. R. (1992). The Zurich study: XIV. Epidemiology of seasonal depression. *European Archives of Psychiatry and Clinical Neuroscience, 241,* 301-306.

Wiggins, C. L., Schmidt-Nowara, W. W., Coultas, D. B., & Samet, J. M. (1990). Comparison of self- and spouse reports of snoring and other symptoms associated with sleep apnea syndrome. *Sleep, 13(3),* 245-252.

Wong, J. L., Regennitter, R. P., & Barrios, F. (1994). Base rate and simulated symptoms of mild head injury among normals. *Archives of Clinical Neuropsychology, 9(5),* 411-425.

Woods, N. F., Most, A., & Dery, G. K. (1982). Prevalence of perimenstrual symptoms. *American Journal of Public Health, 72(11),* 1257-1264.

Yu, M., Hsu, C., Gladen, B., & Rogan, W. J. (1991). In utero PCB/PCDF exposure: Relation of developmental delay to dysmorphology and dose. *Neurotoxicology and Teratology, 13,* 195-202.

Yuk, V. J., Jugdutt, A. V. et al. (1990). "Towards a definition of PMS: A factor analytic evaluation of premenstrual change in non-complaining women." *Journal of Psychosomatic Research* 34(4): 439-446.

Zimmer, J. G., Watson, N. et al. (1984). "Behavioral problems among patients in skilled nursing facilities." *American Journal of Public Health* 74(10): 1118-1121.

Symptom Index